The Key to Medical Literacy

Unlocking the Mysteries of the Physical Exam

By

Neil B. Shulman, M.D.
Edmond Moses, M.D.
Daniel D. Adame, Ph.D

Custom Publisher Kent Hughes
Senior Production Administrator Sue Dunaway

THE KEY TO MEDICAL LITERACY
UNLOCKING THE MYSTERIES OF THE PHYSICAL EXAM

Printed in the United States of America

0-15-503620-3

Biographies

Neil B. Shulman, M.D.

Neil Shulman is an Associate Professor in the Department of Medicine at Emory University in Atlanta, Georgia. He has been co-investigator of research grants in excess of $6 million, and has taught medical students, nursing students and residents for over 20 years. He is an author of 12 books, which include novels, health education books, and children's books. One of his novels, *Doc Hollywood*, was made into a major motion picture starring Michael J. Fox. Dr. Shulman also lectures internationally on a wide variety of serious topics and performs stand-up comedy for charities.

Edmond B. Moses III, M.D.

After graduating from Emory College in 1989 with a degree in Religion, Dr. Moses entered the Emory University School of Medicine and graduated with honors in 1993. It was while at Emory that Dr. Moses recognized the need for the education of patients as informed consumers of medical care, and began to write this book with oversight from his advisor and co-author, Dr. Neil Shulman. Dr. Moses is currently completing his last year of specialization in Family Practice at the Ventura County Medical Center in California.

Daniel D. Adame, Ph.D.

A founding member and former president of the Georgia Federation for Professional Health Educators, Professor Adame is associate professor of health education in the Department of Health and Physical Education at Emory University in Atlanta, Georgia. Dr. Adame teaches and coordinates the health education course which all students are required to take for graduation from Emory College (PE 101). Approximately 1,100 students pass through his classroom each year. A post-doctoral Lilly Teaching Fellow, he was awarded the Emory Williams Excellence in Teaching Award during the Emory College diploma ceremony in the spring of 1994. A member of the Board of Reviewers for *Health Values: The Journal of Health Behavior, Education and Promotion,* Dr. Adame is the author of numerous articles and abstracts centered on his two primary programs of research on "Physical Fitness, Body Image and Locus of Control," and "AIDS Risk Reduction Practices Among Adolescents."

Other Books by Neil Shulman
Summaries

Fiction:
1. ***Finally ... I'm a Doctor***. The funny -- and sometimes autobiographical -- story of a medical student making his way through medical school. *Finally ... I'm a Doctor* is a charming story about a young man and his Jewish grandmother, who gives him lots of advice, from taking an enema once a month to clean his lower bowels, to not loving too much, "you know what I mean". (ISBN #0-938289-32-2)

2. ***Doc Hollywood***. The story of a newly-graduated doctor on a cross-country trip to his future job as a plastic surgeon. His car breaks down in Grady, South Carolina and he's forced to stay there to work off his debt. This book was made into a major motion picture in the United States, starring Michael J. Fox.

3. ***The Backyard Tribe***. This is the story of a doctor on a flying doctor mission in Africa who comes across a little Maasai girl who needs heart surgery. He arranges to bring the little girl to the United States for surgery and the entire tribe accompanies and sets up their village in an upscale Atlanta neighborhood. Walt Disney Studios has developed a screenplay based on the book. (ISBN # 0-312-10513-4)

4. ***Second Wind***. This book contains hilarious adventures of what really goes on in nursing homes -- beauty pageants, romance, fishing expeditions, and more. The nursing home is much more than "God's Waiting Room", in fact, it's the place where many folks catch their second wind. (ISBN # 0-9639002-6-9)

5. ***Life Before Sex.*** Also somewhat autobiographical, this book tells how Neil Barnett and his friends discover the mysterious secrets of growing up. Puberty, they decide, is something to stay away from and make a pact never to grow up. They form a club, the Puberty Prevention Club, and go to great lengths to make sure the Post-Puberty generation understands their message. It is now available in a pre-publication manuscript.

Non-Fiction
1. ***Better Health Care for Less***. An easy-to-use guide with over 350 entries and 1,000 tips on how to save money and improve the quality of your health care. It's full of resources and practical advice that can help you get the information you need on a variety of health conditions. (ISBN # 0-7818-0122-2)

2. ***The Black Man's Guide to Good Health***. This book offers lifesaving information and advice to black men of all ages. Based on the most current medical research, this unique, indispensable reference covers all aspects of black men's health -- from insights on general wellness to important facts about a wide range of illnesses and conditions. (ISBN # 0-399-52138-0)

3. *High Blood Pressure*. Three of America's top experts in the field have put together the latest information on high blood pressure concerning detection, diet, medical tests, drug therapy and drug side effects. (ISBN # 0-440-21693-1)

4. *Understanding Growth Hormone*. This book explains, in layman's terms, the history of growth hormone. Drawing on the latest research as well as on interviews with patients, parents and professionals, the authors review hormone history, give a crash course in endocrinology, visit children whose dreams of normal height are coming true, and delve into the dilemmas and complexities of harnessing the hormone's growth-promoting powers. The book also provides an update on the "fountain of youth" research conducted relating to this hormone. (ISBN # 0-7818-0071-4)

Children's Books

1. *What's in a Doctor's Bag?* explains exactly what those instruments are that the doctor uses in easy to understand language for kids. The story centers around a little boy's trip to the doctor and his hesitation about it. As soon as the doctor closes the door behind him -- Presto! The instruments climb out of the bag, turn into loveable creatures and introduce themselves. (ISBN# 0-9639002-3-4)

2. *Under the Backyard Sky* is a beautifully illustrated account of a little girl named Lucy whose father is a heart surgeon who spends much of his time in Kenya with the Maasai tribe. One day the little girl's father returns home, along with a Maasai girl, Annah, and her whole tribe. Annah needs heart surgery. Lucy has an angry heart because her father spends so much time with the Maasai girl. The Maasai witch doctors get her dad to spend more time with her. *Under the Backyard Sky* is about two little girls, both with broken hearts, and how they become repaired by professionals from other cultures. (ISBN # 1-56145-093-6)

For more information contact:

Neil Shulman
2272 Vistamont Drive
Decatur, GA 30033
Tel: (404) 321-0126
Fax: (404) 633-9198

Acknowledgements

Special recognition to Tim Dignam and Peter Davis for their contributions to the chapter: The Gynecological Exam. Also, to Peter and Tim for the commendable energies they put into writing the Exercise: Practice What You've Learned section. We'd also like to thank those health professionals who have taken the time to read, critique and make valuable suggestions for this book: Dr. Jennifer Hines, Dr. Angela Lee, Arlene Kehir, Dr. Rich Johnson, Dr. Gerald McGorisk, Dr. John Rock, Dr. Charles Wooten and Dr. Lisa Rarick.

Dedication

This book is dedicated to the students of Emory University who have contributed their feedback during the development of this program to help the world become more medically literate. Medical literacy is the missing link in quality health care. We feel that health education is just as important as the three R's, for without health, it's difficult to read, write or do arithmetic.

Illustrations
by

Halcyon Winter
Norbert Schaum
and
Todd Stolp, M.D.

DISCLAIMER

The information in this book is for educational purposes only and is not intended as medical advice. No testing, diagnosis, or treatment should be implemented without consultation with a physician.

NOTICE TO READERS

If you like this book and you are interested in a special, custom-published version of the book indivudualized for your needs, or you would like a specific chapter developed into a brochure, please contact Kent Hughes at Harcourt Brace Custom Publishing, 301 Commerce Street, Suite 3700, Fort Worth, Texas 76102; Tel: (817) 334-7771; Fax: (817) 334-7880.

Table of Contents

CHAPTERS

Table of Illustrations

The pages in this book are perforated so that readers may remove and use selected sections at their discretion.

Chapter 1

What's in a Doctor's Bag?

This book was written for the purpose of educating you about what doctors learn from conducting a physical examination of the human body so that you can play an active role with your physician, rather than a passive one often shrouded by mystique, anxiety and fear. Whether or not you've ever had a complete physical examination, this book can help you better understand your body and what doctors learn from their examining procedures.

In spite of the fact that our bodies are the very vehicles that get us around and through which we experience life, many people know or understand little about their bodies. The first line of defense against illness is an educated consumer who knows his or her body and is sensitive to any bodily changes that are not normal.

Almost without exception, every disease is characterized by certain physical findings. Thus, assessing the human body through the physical examination is of utmost importance to determine what is going on. While in today's world of high tech medicine the physical examination may seem to take a back seat to other types of exams and tests, a good physician will always complete a thorough physical examination before proceeding with any other tests.

The contents of this book will help explain to the reader what exactly is going on in the mind of the physician while she or he conducts the physical examination. The chapters in this book will explain, in simple terms, what the physician is looking at, listening to, feeling or tapping on, in the various parts of the patient's body.

In today's world, people want to know increasingly more about the things which pertain to their health. But with medical advances being made almost daily, people are being left further and further behind. Typically, there is a large communication gap between the physician and patient, since physicians speak in what is, to most, a foreign language. Countless patients are frustrated by the lack of understandable communication from their physicians about their problems and proposed treatment. Patients want to know what the doctor was thinking, what he or she learned from the examination, and why a particular course of treatment was prescribed.

The chapters in this book will explain the importance of the physical examination, and which basic methods and instruments are used by the physician to examine the body. Each major organ system will be covered by a chapter. Interspersed throughout the book are interesting suggestions and experiments designed to challenge the reader to learn more about the human body by looking, listening, feeling and tapping. At long last will be explained the use of those mysterious instruments contained in the doctor's black bag!

Becoming medically literate has its advantages. For example, did you know that if a person accidentally falls and injures his head, a simple examination that can be performed very quickly could possibly save his life? Indeed, when looking into this person's eyes, if one pupil is larger than the other, this could indicate that there may be serious brain injury. This person should be brought to an emergency room as soon as possible. Yet another example is one in which a person complains of a serious headache. If this individual cannot lower their head to touch their chest, she or he might have a disease called meningitis. This too is a condition that should receive immediate medical attention. Bringing this to a doctor's attention could result in starting intravenous antibiotics, a procedure which could save this person's life. Finally, do you know the symptoms of appendicitis? Which side of the body would this affect? More specifically, in which quadrant of the abdomen would one detect tenderness?

Don't be overly disturbed if, as a consequence of learning more about your body and the various diseases discussed in this book, you begin to feel you might have one of these illnesses. Chances are, you don't! As a matter of fact, you might be interested in learning that many medical students go through phases in which they become convinced they are ill with some of the diseases they are studying. In most cases, the student is only over-sensitive. Of course, if you do notice an abnormal finding, check with your doctor.

SO WHAT'S IN THE DOCTOR'S BAG?

The following is a brief description of the instruments included in the doctor's bag and what they are used for when examining the body.

The Ophthalmoscope: The ophthalmoscope is an optical instrument used for looking inside the eyes. It is made up of a system of lenses and mirrors that enables the doctor to see the various internal structures. A light source inside the instrument provides illumination. Through the regulation of different size openings in the instrument, the doctor can control the amount of light entering the eye. The lenses, of various powers of magnification, are used to bring the structures being examined into focus.

The Otoscope: The otoscope is an instrument used to examine the ear canal and ear drum. The speculum, which comes in various sizes, is placed in the ear canal. An attached glass plate serves as a viewing window and a magnifying glass. The otoscope and ophthalmoscope use the same base which serves as a handle and usually contains a battery to power the light source.

Stethoscope: The stethoscope is used for listening to sounds inside the body (eg: the heart, the lungs, and the bowels). Sound waves are transmitted along the rubber tubing of the stethoscope to the earpieces. The end piece has two components: one is called the diaphragm, which is flat, and the other has the shape of a bell. The diaphragm screens out low pitched sounds and transmits high pitched sounds. The bell endpiece utilizes the skin of the patient as a diaphragm. So, depending on the amount of pressure exerted by the doctor on the bell, the pitch of the sounds heard will vary. Generally, the bell is best for hearing low-pitched sounds.

Reflex Hammer: In examining the nervous system, the doctor uses the padded reflex hammer which has a pointed and a flat end. Gently striking various points on the body, the physician is able to test deep tendon reflexes.

Blood Pressure Cuff: The blood pressure cuff, when used along with the stethoscope, is utilized to measure a patient's blood pressure. The blood pressure instrument is made up of an inflatable cuff that is designed to go around an upper arm, a pressure meter, and a rubber hand bulb with a pressure control valve which is used to inflate and deflate the rubber cuff. After placing the cuff around the upper arm, the doctor inflates the cuff. As air exits the inflated cuff (released through the control valve), blood more easily passes through an artery that runs along the inside of the elbow. With the stethoscope in place, the doctor hears the blood pass through and records the blood pressure, while observing the pressure meter.

Thermometer: Measurement of the body temperature provides important information as to the severity of a patient's illness. Mercury thermometers have long been used in taking temperatures by mouth, under the arm, or rectally. Today, modern technology has produced an electronic thermometer that can be used to measure the body temperature through the ear. Using infrared technology, a temperature reading is available in two seconds.

Tongue Depressor: The tongue depressor is used to look inside the mouth. Depressing the tongue and having the patient say "ahh" clears the view in back of the throat, enabling the doctor to inspect the tonsils and the back of the throat.

CHAPTER 2

The Patient's History

Taking a history from a patient is the single most important interaction that occurs between doctor and patient. The history is a description of the events and conditions that led to the patient feeling sick and seeking medical assistance.

It includes the condition for which the patient may have come to the doctor, as well as any previous illnesses or medical conditions that may be relevant to the present problem. It is the history that gives the most useful information for the doctor and gives the best clue of what is troubling the patient. In fact, the history is so important that correctly obtaining and recording it is an art in itself. It is not just asking a series of questions, but also recognizing subtleties such as the patient's demeanor, which may reveal unspoken concerns.

When certain disease processes are suspected, doctors are taught to ask relevant questions in a certain order and manner. This order and manner standardizes the recording of the history which allows for easier and more consistent communication between doctors.

For example, the history is often recorded in the following manner:

Chief Complaint: this is the main concern that troubles the patient and is usually stated in the patient's own words.

History of Present Illness: this records the chronological order of the patient's symptoms and complaints as the patient remembers them. This should begin with the first symptom or disturbance that was noticed and the day and time when it occurred. This should be followed by a story of all that has happened in the mean time, up to and including the day of the appointment to see the doctor.

Past Medical and Surgical History: this should include all significant past medical information that the patient provides, as well as any surgery that has been performed and also if there were any complications during the surgical procedures.

Medications: this should include all medicines being taken by the patient at present, including non-prescription drugs. All drugs taken in the last six months should also be included.

Allergies: this should include all drug allergies and previous drug reactions (including exactly what reaction occurred) as well as any known food allergies.

Social History: this part of the patient's history includes the patient's profession, marital status, living arrangements, and whether or not the patient smokes, consumes alcohol, coffee, or uses illegal drugs. It is also important to question everyone regarding risk factors for contracting diseases such as hepatitis (inflammation of the liver) and Human Immuno-deficiency Virus (HIV, the virus that causes AIDS), as well as other sexually transmitted diseases (STDs).

Review of the Body's Systems: this is a mental checklist that a doctor keeps in mind and reviews with the patient. It contains several questions that are related to each major organ system of the body and allows a quick assessment of the overall health and well-being of a patient. For example, in reviewing the pulmonary system (lungs) a doctor might ask if the patient has been exposed to tuberculosis or had other lung diseases such as asthma. Many of the questions in a complete review of the body's systems are good for screening about diseases that may have gone unnoticed by the patient.

This recorded list completes a thorough history. Obviously, such a thorough history is not taken every time a patient comes to the doctor, but complete histories are always recommended the first time a patient is seen by a new doctor or whenever a patient is being admitted to the hospital. When a doctor sees a patient for a relatively uncomplicated problem, it is often not necessary to be so complete. The chief complaint and history of the current illness are usually sufficient.

A. The Importance of the Physical Exam: Second in importance only to taking a history from the patient is the physician's examination of the patient. Simply by looking at a person a skilled physician will often be able to quickly assess how sick the patient really is, and, after completing a thorough physical examination, the doctor should have a good idea about what the diagnosis is. In fact, if the history and physical examination does not leave the doctor with a pretty good idea about what is going on, it is often unlikely that additional expensive laboratory tests and diagnostic studies will be of much use.

Conducting the physical examination is much like taking the history. Doctors are required to learn very detailed ways of examining the body and to know the difference between what is normal and what is not normal. The physical examination is conducted in a particular order and each major organ system is examined separately. Most doctors prefer to use the same order in examining each patient so that no important parts of the exam are left out. The order most often followed goes from head to foot.

The physical examination itself will not be discussed any further at this point since it is the subject of the rest of the book, but suffice it to say that a doctor needs to examine each patient carefully and thoroughly on each visit. Remember, when a doctor sees one of his or her regular patients for an uncomplicated and common problem (like a cold), it may not be necessary to conduct a complete physical examination each time. The doctor may choose to make the examination shorter and perform only those parts that are relevant to the patient's complaint at that time.

B. The Doctor's Methods: When performing the physical exam, there are several methods of observation which doctors have been trained to use in a particular order. These methods involve the use of the doctor's eyes, ears, and sense of touch. Each of these methods provides different types of information, all of which are useful in determining what the problem is. For each of these a doctor must know what is normal, what is abnormal, and learn to judge what might be wrong when abnormal findings are noticed.

1. Looking (Inspection): One of the most valuable tools that a doctor has is simply looking at the patient. A doctor's eyes provide him or her with a wealth of information which cannot be gained in any other way. As you know, doctors are often unwilling to treat people "over the phone" and the reason for this is a good one -- without seeing the patient, much less information can be gathered about the patient's condition.

Doctors are taught to carefully inspect the patient's body. The obvious places that need to be seen are the skin, the hair and the nails -- each can reveal clues as to the cause or presence of certain disease processes. A doctor must also, at certain times, carefully inspect each of the openings to the body, such as the mouth, ears or anus. The observation skills of a doctor are important, for example, when a doctor is examining the chest and lungs of a patient, it will be important to observe the movements of the chest wall during breathing and to see which of the muscles for breathing the patient is using. It is also important to observe whether or not the chest wall is symmetrical and moves equally on both sides while breathing.

Finally, and probably the most important observation that the doctor makes, is the overall appearance and condition of a patient. People, whether they know it or not, reveal a great deal about themselves just by the way they dress and groom, and by the way they behave in certain situations (for example: sitting, talking, walking). Doctors are trained to pick up on these clues and to use each observation to form a more accurate view of the patient. Usually, an experienced doctor is able to accurately assess how sick a person really is just by observing them for a few minutes. This overall assessment is an art which is not only perfected through years of experience, but is essential to good clinical judgement. The next time you visit your doctor, remember that by the time you have finished telling him or her what is wrong, she or he has not only been listening to you, but has also been gathering additional information by observing even the finest details about your appearance and the way your body looks.

2. Listening (Auscultation): Listening is probably the second most valuable tool of examination that the doctor uses. If you consider how important listening to the patient's complaint and history is, then listening is, by far, the most important tool which the doctor has. But here, we are referring especially to the type of listening that doctors call "auscultation". Doctors use stethoscopes on a daily basis to listen to the body's internal organs. A stethoscope is the instrument which the doctor places in his ears while placing the other end on a part of the body to listen. What cannot be seen can often be heard, so doctors spend much time at the end of a stethoscope listening to what is going on inside. Most of us know that doctors use stethoscopes to listen to the heart to hear if it is beating normally, and to hear whether there are any abnormal sounds present. Many of us have probably had a doctor put a stethoscope to our chest and ask us to breathe deeply. Here, the doctor is listening to the lungs. These two uses of the stethoscope are invaluable to the doctor in making an assessment and have never been replaced by any modern technology or test.

Other uses of the stethoscope involve listening over certain blood vessels in the head, neck, abdomen and groin to see if there are any abnormal "swooshing" sounds which indicate that blood is flowing unevenly around diseased arteries or veins. Doctors also frequently listen to the abdomen to hear what sounds the intestines are making (bowel sounds). We have all heard our stomachs grumble from time to time, but actually our stomachs and intestines are constantly moving (called peristalsis) and making faint noises that we usually cannot hear. Doctors use these sounds to help determine if the intestines are blocked, irritated, or moving much faster or slower than usual. If you put your ear to someone's stomach and listen carefully for about 30 seconds, you will hear noises which are probably caused by the normal movement of the intestines.

3. Feeling (Palpation): There are many sayings about the doctor's hands which emphasize the importance of touch in the diagnostic and healing process. What cannot be seen or heard can often be felt, and it is for this reason that a doctor's fingers and hands are of such use to him or her. Doctors use their sense of touch daily, especially in examining the head and neck, the heart, the chest and lungs, and the abdomen. In addition, the hands are often used to help examine the arms and legs, the sex organs, and even the inside of the mouth or rectum.

The hands are often used in combination with the visual inspection which the doctor does. In fact, almost everything that appears abnormal requires an examination by palpation because it will often feel abnormal as well. For example, if the doctor sees an unusual red spot in the mouth of a person being examined, the next step is to feel for consistency (how hard or soft it is). This will give clues that help the doctor to decide whether the spot is a tumor (abnormal growth) or just an irritated area, and whether further tests are needed.

In general, doctors should carefully palpate all abnormal growths and try to determine three things: (1) whether the tumor is soft, firm, or very hard; (2) whether the tumor is solid, fluid-filled, or hollow (cystic) (3) whether the tumor is attached to the tissue below it, or whether it moves freely.

Feeling can sometimes be uncomfortable for the patient. When a doctor conducts an examination which requires palpation, remember that this palpation is an important part of the information being gathered. By taking the time to feel carefully, a doctor is providing you with the best care and trying to avoid expensive and unnecessary tests and procedures.

4. Tapping (Percussion): Tapping (or percussing) is done less today than in years past because today we have technology available which provides much of the same information which tapping provided to doctors many years ago, and with much more accuracy. By tapping on or over an organ, a doctor is trying to determine the relative similarity of the organ or tissue being percussed as compared to the organs of other patients. Percussion is done in a fairly specific manner: the middle finger of one hand is placed over the area being examined while the middle and index fingers of the other hand are used to tap firmly several times. The sounds produced are described as being either dull, flat or tympanic. Dull is the sound made when tapping over a relatively hollow organ such as the lungs or intestines. Flat is the sound heard when tapping over a solid organ such as the liver or kidneys. Try tapping on someone's back. Start up at one of the lungs and see if you can hear a dull sound, then move downward as you continue tapping and see if you can tell where the sound becomes flat. If you can, you have identified where the lung ends. If, for example, the bottom part of the lung was partially filled with fluid (as in pneumonia) you might hear the flat sound higher up in the chest than normal and suspect that there must be an abnormal collection of fluid there. Tympanitic percussion is the sound that you hear over areas where there is air which is under pressure. This is normally not heard, but may be present when the abdomen is abnormally distended with air, or when air has collected under pressure inside the chest wall, but outside of the lungs.

Percussion is used primarily in examining the lungs and abdomen. It is generally useful for determining the size and amount of expansion of the lungs, as well as whether or not there are collections of fluid around the lungs. Percussion is most useful during the abdominal exam when estimating the size of the liver and spleen.

CHAPTER 3

The Vital Signs

Often, the very first thing which will be done to examine your body is to record your vital signs. There are four signs that are easy to measure which give a large amount of important information: heart rate (pulse), rate of breathing (respirations), blood pressure, and body temperature. Usually, the vital signs are taken by a nurse or medical technician in the waiting area before your physician sees you and are recorded for the doctor to review.

The vital signs are measurements which are easily recognized and interpreted by all medical personnel. They provide a quick assessment of how sick someone is and how urgently they need medical care. This is especially useful in the emergency room where patients are treated according to who is in need of the most urgent care and not on a first-come, first-serve basis. For example, someone with a very high heart rate and a very low blood pressure could be bleeding internally and require immediate attention.

If a person is critically ill and in danger of dying, he or she should be seen and treated before someone who has a sprained ankle. This priority system for treating patients (called "triage") is not always popular with the patients who have to wait.

By looking at vital signs, a doctor can tell whether the patient is "stable" and will not be harmed by waiting, or "unstable" and in need of immediate life-saving measures. The vital signs are also an inexpensive way to screen for a wide variety of medical diseases.

All screening tests have advantages and disadvantages. The advantages are that taking the vital signs is quick, painless and cheap. The major disadvantage is that the information obtained is often very general and rarely gives the specific cause of the problem. In other words, the vital signs are good at telling if something serious is going on, but usually not too good at telling exactly what is wrong.

1. Heart Rate and Rhythm: In assessing the beating of the heart, there are two primary concerns: the rate at which the heart is beating and the rhythm with which the heart beats. We all know that the heart's function is to pump blood to the rest of the body in order to supply oxygen and nutrients while removing carbon dioxide and other wastes. It makes sense, therefore, that the faster the heart is beating, the more blood is being pumped to the body. Conversely, the opposite is also true.

Certain heart rates can be dangerous. If the heart is beating too slowly there is a danger that the body will not get enough oxygen and nutrients, or that it will not be able to remove enough carbon dioxide and other wastes. On the other hand, if the heart is beating too fast, the pump is having to work too hard and may need more oxygen than can be supplied. This places parts of the heart muscle in danger of dying from lack of oxygen.

What is a normal, resting heart rate? That depends on the person's age. It is said that the normal adult heart rate is 72-80 beats per minute. This is true for most resting adults; however, children have heart rates which are faster than adults and a newborn baby has a normal, resting heart rate of 120-160 beats per minute! Athletes who are in good physical condition may have a normal heart rate of 50-60.

The maximum safe heart rate is an important concept because at rates above this safe maximum the heart can be in great danger. The highest safe heart rate is determined by the formula: person's age subtracted from 220 = maximum safe heart rate. It is also helpful to know that the heart rate which is best for beneficial aerobic exercise is 75-80% of the maximum safe heart rate. There is no set minimum safe heart rate, but slow heart rates are determined to be normal or not, based on associated symptoms. If a person with a slow heart rate feels weak and tired, their heart rate may not be fast enough to pump blood to their entire body (this could also be due to a blood pressure which is too low).

In extreme circumstances, a very slow heart rate will cause a person to lose consciousness because the brain is not receiving enough oxygen to "stay awake".

Some Factors Which Increase Heart Rate:

1. Body temperature: In general, the heart rate increases 10 beats per minute for every one degree Fahrenheit which the body temperature increases. So, a person with a fever will have a faster heart rate than a person without a fever.

2. Anxiety: When a person is afraid, the nervous system is more aroused than normal and is preparing for any emergency that might come along. The brain sends signals to the heart to make it beat faster so the body will have enough oxygen to respond to any situation.

3. Pain: Pain generally increases a person's anxiety level, thereby causing the heart rate to increase.

4. Exercise: Any person who is exercising is using more oxygen and producing more carbon dioxide than they are when resting, so they need more blood flowing in their body to meet these increased demands. Naturally, the heart rate increases to help supply the extra blood that is needed by the rest of the body.

5. Hyperthyroidism: The thyroid gland is a gland located below the Adam's apple in the neck. It secretes hormones that determine how much and how fast energy is used by the body. This is called the body's metabolic rate and it is mostly determined by the level of thyroid hormone in the blood. If this hormonal level rises, as it can with some diseases, it causes the body to accelerate all of its functions including the heart rate.

6. Anemia: Anemia is when there are not enough red blood cells in the blood to carry oxygen to the body, and is caused by many diseases. In this condition the heart compensates by pumping more blood and therefore, the heart rate increases.

7. Medications: Many medications increase the heart rate, either directly by acting on the heart itself, or indirectly by affecting the brain or other organs.

Some Factors Which Decrease the Heart Rate:

1. Sleep/Rest: Sleeping people generally have heart rates that are slower than when they are awake. Taking the pulse of someone who lives in your house while they are sitting in front of the television and then taking it again after they go to sleep will prove this point.

2. Organic Heart Disease: The heart rate is regulated by electric signals which come from the top of the heart and spread out along special channels to all of the heart muscle. When the heart muscle becomes damaged or diseased, the signal for it to beat may not be generated or may be improperly transmitted, causing the rate to slow down.

3. Hypothyroidism: In the same way that too much thyroid hormone can speed up the body's metabolic rate, too little hormone from the thyroid gland can slow down the metabolic rate so much that the heart slows down also.

4. Medications: Many medications can slow down the heart rate. In fact, many of the medicines used to treat irregular heart rhythms also have the effect of slowing the heart.

TAKING THE PULSE:

Where on my body can my doctor feel my pulse and why would she or he want to feel it in different places? There are many places where the pulse can be felt, but the most common is the wrist. Others sites include: beside the eyes in the temples, in the neck to either side of the trachea (wind-pipe), under the arm, in the fold of the elbow, in the groin, behind the knee, on top of the feet, and on the inside of the ankle just below where the bone of the shin ends. **[Figure 3A]**

The easiest place to take the pulse is to feel for it on the wrist. To take the heart rate, press over the correct places with the pad of your index and middle finger until you feel pulsations. Count the number of beats that you feel in one minute, or count the number of beats that you feel in 15 seconds and multiply this by four to get the rate per minute. Do not use your thumb since it has a pulse of its own which is often felt.

Feeling the pulse at the same place on both sides of the body tells the doctor that the arteries on both sides are the same and that both have blood flowing through them.

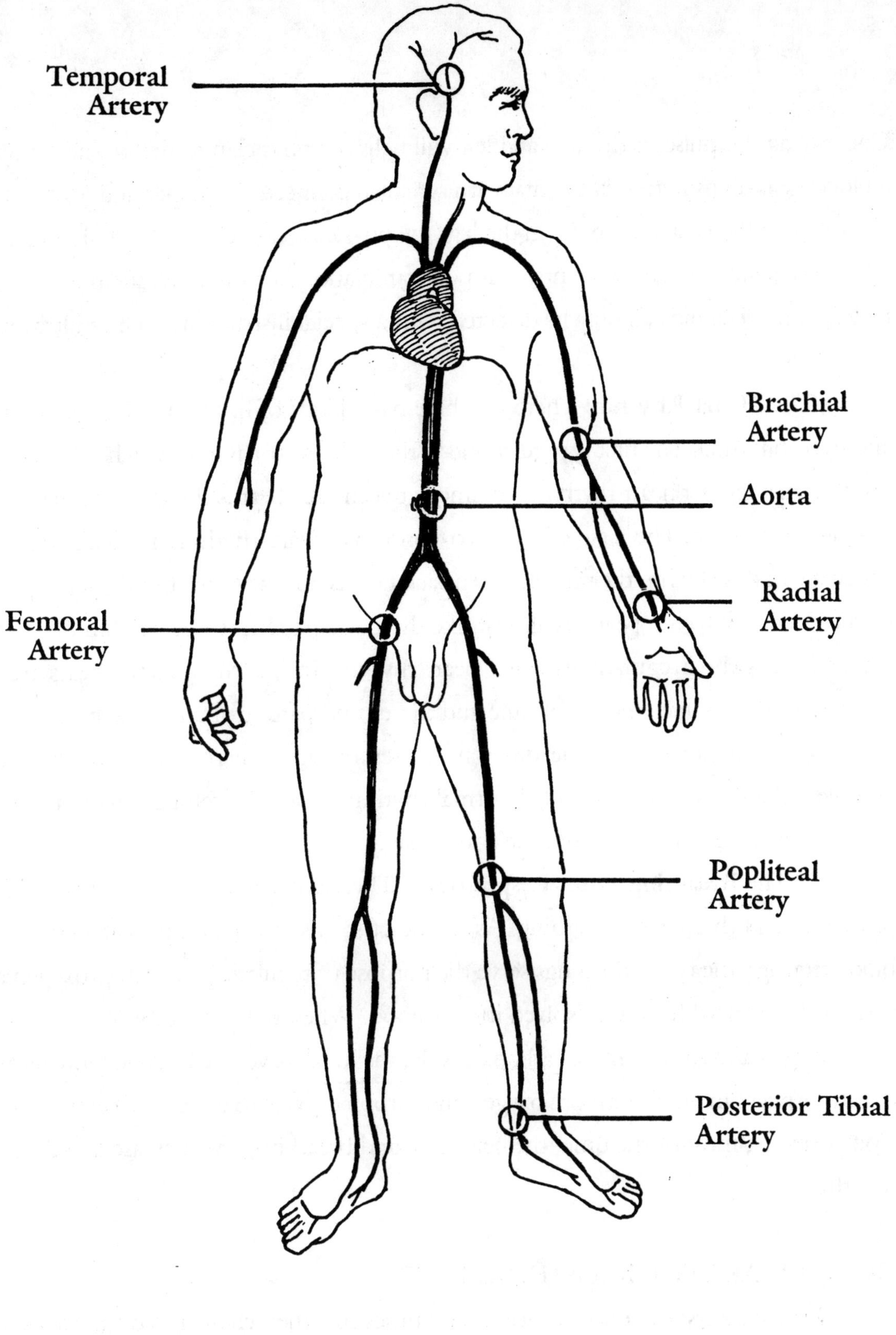

FEELING THE PULSES

Figure 3A

Comparing the pulse in the arm and leg will help the physician to determine if there is a blockage or constriction in the main artery which connects the upper and lower halves of the body. By feeling the pulse in the legs the physician can tell if the circulation in the feet is adequate. In many patients with poor circulation, for example, the pulses cannot be felt in the feet and can only be detected with a special instrument such as ultrasound.

The Heart Rhythm: There are three basic kinds of heart rhythms: one normal and two abnormal. The first is regular and is the only heart rhythm which is considered normal. In a regular heart rhythm, the time between each beat is the same, similar to the ticking of a clock. The first of the two abnormal heart rhythms is called regularly irregular. In this rhythm the time between each beat is not the same, but there is a pattern to the rhythm which repeats itself, just like there is a pattern to the rhythm of a waltz. Next, there is the irregularly irregular heart rhythm. In this rhythm, the beats are not separated by the same amount of time and there is no pattern at all to the beats.

We will not discuss the different causes of all these rhythms, which is very complex. Suffice it to say that all abnormal rhythms deserve careful evaluation because they can be dangerous; however, most are treatable.

2. The Breathing Rate (Respiration): There are many similarities between the heart rate and the rate of breathing. As the heart serves as the pump which moves the blood through the body, the lungs serve the purpose of regulating the gases (oxygen and carbon dioxide) which are dissolved in the blood. When the heart beats fast to supply more oxygen and remove more carbon dioxide, the lungs have to exchange more air with the atmosphere in order for more oxygen and carbon dioxide to enter and leave the body. Consequently, most of the time, the heart rate and breathing rate increase and decrease together.

HOW TO TAKE THE BREATHING RATE:

Watch a person breathe and count the times that their chest rises during a minute. You can also count the times the chest rises during 15 seconds and multiply by four just as you did with the heart rate. It is often important that the person not know that you are counting each breath because they will become aware of their breathing and their breathing rate will usually increase. Experienced nurses will count the breathing rate during the pulse or temperature measurement, without the patient ever knowing that this is going on.

So what is a normal breathing rate, and what controls the rate at which one breathes? It is said that a normal adult with healthy lungs breathes 12-20 times a minute. Just as the normal heart rate is faster in children, so is the normal breathing rate. There are two factors which control the amount of air which is exchanged with the atmosphere: the level of oxygen in the blood and the level of carbon dioxide in the blood. Both of these levels are sensed by the brain on a minute to minute basis and adjustments are made in the rate and depth of breathing to keep these levels constant.

A person breathes in oxygen and exhales carbon dioxide. Without this oxygen our brain and other organs would not be able to function. After the oxygen is used by the body, it is turned into carbon dioxide, which is an acid, and should not stay in the body. In order for the carbon dioxide to be exhaled, the acid must cross over from the blood back into the lungs and out of the body.

The exhalation of carbon dioxide from the body to clear the blood of acid build-up is the main factor which controls our rate of breathing -- the higher the level of carbon dioxide, the faster we breathe to remove it. At the rate of breathing which gets rid of enough carbon dioxide, we are already moving enough air into and out of our lungs to provide adequate oxygen. Thus, the oxygen level in our blood does not directly control our rate of breathing. However, in people with certain lung diseases (i.e. emphysema), enough acid has built up in their bodies that their brain has begun to ignore carbon dioxide as a stimulus to breathe. These people have a rate of breathing which is controlled directly by the level of oxygen in their blood -- when the level gets low, they breathe faster.

There is no set maximum or minimum safe rate of breathing. A person who is exercising vigorously may breathe 40-50 times per minute, while one who is asleep may breathe 10-12 times per minute. It is true, however, that the faster you breathe, the more energy it takes to breathe and the more tired your muscles for breathing will become. A person who is breathing extremely fast is in danger of tiring out his or her muscles for breathing, and may stop breathing altogether. On the other hand, a person who is breathing too slowly is likely not getting rid of enough acid and may not even be supplying the blood with enough oxygen.

Some factors which increase the breathing rate:

Many of the factors which increase the heart rate also increase the breathing rate, such as anxiety, fever, pain, exercise and hyperthyroidism.

In addition, diseases which cause the body to produce more acid require an increased rate of breathing to rid the body of the extra acid. These include uncontrolled diabetes, kidney disease, infection, ingestion of certain poisons, drug overdosing, starvation, diarrhea, sickle cell anemia and many others.

Some factors which decrease the breathing rate:

Many of the factors which decrease the heart rate also decrease the breathing rate, such as sleep and certain medications. Many drugs, such as powerful pain killers and alcohol, can reduce the rate of breathing to dangerously low rates.

When the lungs move less air in and out, acid builds up in the blood. Usually, this is not good; however, this can be used by the body to make up for when there is not enough acid in the blood. For instance, while vomiting causes a person to lose a significant amount of stomach acid, the body can slow the rate of breathing, thereby increasing the amount of acid in the blood. Additional factors which decrease the rate of breathing include excess of certain body hormones, excessive antacid ingestion, kidney failure and even some cancers.

Rhythm and depth of breathing: It is normal to breathe with regular rhythm and to take breaths at regular intervals. Big breaths and small breaths generally waste too much energy and are not an efficient way of exchanging gas into and out of the lungs. For this reason the brain regulates both the rate and the depth of breathing to control the total amount of air which the lungs use.

In certain diseases or injuries the rhythm of breathing can be altered significantly. For example, when a person has fractured some ribs and the bones are poking into the lungs, it hurts to breathe. Naturally, the brain compensates and the breathing becomes shallow to decrease the pain, but faster to keep the total volume of air exchanged the same. Other abnormal rhythms are seen in certain head injuries when patients usually breathe both rapidly and deeply.

Finally, here's a quick way which doctors use to determine how much energy a person is using to breathe. The diaphragm (a powerful muscle which separates the chest from the abdomen) is responsible for most of the effort of breathing. When a person needs to breathe faster and deeper, other muscles join in to help. These include the abdominal muscles, some of the muscles in between the ribs, and some of the neck muscles. Together, these are called the accessory muscles of breathing, and when they are being used, they may indicate that the diaphragm is having to work very hard to breathe and, with prolonged use, it may stop altogether. People cannot breathe for long periods of time with their accessory muscles, and need rapid treatment to assist them in breathing more easily. However, some patients with chronic lung diseases (such as emphysema) may have extra-strong accessory muscles, and are able to use them for extended periods without stopping breathing altogether.

3. The Blood Pressure: Remember that the heart, which is a muscle composed of four chambers, pumps blood to supply oxygen and nutrients to the body while the lungs remove carbon dioxide and other wastes from the body. The heart pumps blood in two different circuits, one of which is under high pressure and one of which is under low pressure. The left side of the heart pumps blood to most of the body and powers the high pressure circuit. The right side of the heart pumps blood to the lungs and powers the low pressure circuit.

In measuring the blood pressure the doctor is measuring the pressure in the high pressure circuit. The blood pressure is recorded as two numbers: one which is usually greater than one hundred, and one usually less than one hundred. For example, a typical adult blood pressure would be 120/80. The top number is called the systolic pressure and the bottom number is called the diastolic pressure. Usually the blood pressure is measured in the arm, using a blood pressure cuff (sphygmomanometer) and stethoscope. It can also be measured at both the thigh and calf.

The high number of the blood pressure measures the pressure in the arteries during the peak of the heart's contraction (while blood is pumped out of the left side of the heart), the low number measures the pressure in the arteries while the heart is resting. The pressure in the arteries is always somewhere in between the high and low numbers and never falls to zero. This constant pressure causes the blood to move forward without stopping.

The heart needs to generate enough pressure to adequately supply the body because too little pressure will cause the blood to move so slowly that organs will not function properly. Too much pressure causes the heart to work harder and can even cause "blowouts" in some of the vessels or heart failure. In some kinds of strokes, brain tissue is damaged when blood vessels burst under high pressure. The brain regulates blood pressure minute by minute by causing the arteries and veins to either clamp down or relax, thereby regulating the body's blood pressure. The pressure can also be altered by the rate and the force of the heart beat.

In assessing the blood pressure as one of the vital signs, only very high and very low pressures are of immediate concern. However, the blood pressure measurement also doubles as a screening test for people with unknown, long-standing high blood pressure, which is not immediately dangerous but needs to be treated.

High Blood Pressure: When a patient has a diastolic blood pressure (the lower number) which is greater than 90 on multiple recordings, treatment is usually necessary. If the systolic blood pressure (the higher number) is repeatedly measured to be greater than 160, treatment is also usually necessary. Patients with untreated high blood pressures are more likely to experience heart attacks, strokes, and kidney failure.

Dangerously Low Blood Pressure: Generally, low blood pressure without the symptoms of weakness or dizziness, is not a problem. When a person is sick, however, their blood pressure can become so dangerously low that their organs do not get enough blood. Very low blood pressure may cause people to feel dizzy and even to faint. When the blood pressure is this low, the brain is not getting enough oxygen to stay awake and the kidneys are not getting blood to produce enough urine.

Causes of Dangerously Low Blood Pressure Include:

Blood loss: When a person is bleeding, there is a hole in the bloodstream and blood is leaking out. If a person has lost a lot of blood, even if they are bleeding internally, the body is unable to compensate for this pressure leak and the blood pressure goes down.

Dehydration: If a person has not taken in enough fluids, they begin to lose too much fluid through their urine, stool, breath, and skin. This can cause the blood pressure to drop.

Heart attack and heart failure: When part of the heart muscle dies after a heart attack, or when the heart is fatigued from pumping under very high pressure, it begins to fail and cannot squeeze hard enough to generate the pressure needed. This causes the blood pressure to drop.

Irregular heart rates: A heart which is beating very slowly fails to generate adequate pressure. Similarly, a very fast beating heart, or a heart beating with a very irregular rhythm, is inefficient and unable to generate adequate pressure. This can cause a low blood pressure.

Drugs, medicines: Many medicines decrease the blood pressure and if overdoses of these medicines are taken they can decrease the blood pressure to dangerously low levels.

Measuring the blood pressure in both arms: Sometimes the blood pressure is measured in both arms in the same way the pulse is sometimes taken in both arms. If there is a big difference between the two, this could mean that there is a narrowing in one of the main arteries. Occasionally the blood pressure is measured in one arm and in one leg. If the difference is large, this could mean that there is a narrowing in the body's largest artery, the aorta.

A person's blood pressure may change from lying down to sitting up or standing. Your doctor will occasionally ask that your blood pressure be taken in the lying, sitting and standing positions. When you sit or stand up, more of your blood collects in your arms and legs, which causes a brief decrease in blood pressure. The brain usually senses this and squeezes down on these vessels so that more blood returns to the heart and the blood pressure goes back up to normal. So normally, one's blood pressure should remain relatively stable when measured in these different positions. In some illnesses, and when a patient is dehydrated or has lost blood, her or his blood pressure might be normal when laying down. However, once the patient sits up and gravity pulls blood into her or his legs, the blood pressure will drop. Because the patient already has a decreased amount of blood in her or his vessels, the brain is unable to compensate enough and the blood pressure remains low and the heart rate goes up. When a person's blood pressure goes down and stays down (or their heart rate goes up more than about 15 beats per minute when moved from lying to sitting), this may mean that the patient's blood volume is low and she or he may need either fluids or blood.

4. Body Temperature: It has long been said that the normal human body temperature is 98.6 degrees Fahrenheit. However, recent studies have shown that a person's normal body temperature can be as high as 99.9 degrees Fahrenheit. Body temperature normally fluctuates over a 24 hour cycle and is lowest at four in the morning and highest at six o'clock in the evening. Body temperature is closely regulated by the brain. In cold conditions the brain speeds up the body's metabolism, causing it to generate more heat. In warm conditions the heat generated by the body's normal metabolism is released by the body in special ways. For example, the skin begins to sweat and this causes cooling. Also, more blood is sent to the skin where the heat can be released.

HOW TO TAKE THE TEMPERATURE:

To record the temperature, a thermometer (either mercury or electric) is placed in close contact with the body for several minutes. The temperature is then read off the scale or meter. Body temperature can be measured in several places: the mouth, under the arm, in the ear, and in the rectum.

The most accurate measurement of body temperature is the rectum since this is completely inside the body. A rectal temperature of greater than 100.5 is generally said to be a fever. When the temperature is taken in the mouth it is generally 0.7 degrees lower than the rectal temperature. When it is taken under the arm, it is generally 1.0 degree lower than the rectal temperature. Remember that normal body temperature is a range and not a specific number.

Causes of high temperatures (fevers): Vigorous exercise (like long distance running) can cause the body temperature to increase two to three degrees Fahrenheit. In addition, many illnesses cause fever. These include infections, tumors, connective tissue diseases (such as rheumatoid arthritis), and drugs. Because fever is such a general sign and has many causes, it is a good indicator that something is wrong but does not accurately indicate what is wrong. Most often fever is a sign of infection of some sort.

When the body has a higher than normal temperature (fever), it does not mean that the brain has stopped regulating body temperature and that things are out of control. What has happened is that the body has reset its own thermostat and is still regulating the temperature, but at a different level.

Some scientists think that by raising its temperature the body is better able to fight off disease, and that germs have a more difficult time growing at higher temperatures.

Another function of fever is obvious -- it makes you feel miserable so you go to bed and get some rest, which could help you recover.

Very high fevers, such as fevers greater than 104 degrees, can be dangerous. When the body temperature is elevated, certain chemical reactions do not occur at their normal rate because the enzymes that control them are partially inactivated by very high temperatures. This means that people with a fever have limitations in their body's normal functions which explains why a fever causes a person to feel weak and achy. Children with high fevers, in addition to being affected by decreased body function, are also at risk for having seizures and so their bodies are often cooled artificially with cool water to prevent seizures.

Causes of low body temperature:

A body temperature below 96 degrees is abnormally low. The most common cause of low body temperature is exposure to cold weather. Here too, the body's enzymes do not function effectively and chemical reactions are slowed. This condition responds well by warming with blankets and is usually not a very big problem.

5. The Level of Oxygen in the Blood (Pulse Oximetry):

For many years there were only four vital signs, however, modern technology has developed a simple way of measuring the oxygen content of the blood. This measurement is called pulse oximetry and is done by placing a light sensing device on the finger of the patient. The light shines into the finger and detects each heart beat and is also able to tell how much oxygen is being carried in the blood. This is especially useful in patients with asthma, emphysema, and pneumonia who may have difficulty getting enough oxygen into their blood. Normally, the hemoglobin in the blood is 95-99% saturated with oxygen. When the lungs are diseased, or when breathing is inadequate, this level can drop to 60 or 70%. It is important to know this, so that adequate treatment can be given and so that it may be determined whether that treatment is working. Pulse oximetry is so simple and accurate that it is being used more often and is being considered by some as the new fifth vital sign.

CHAPTER 4

The Ears, Nose and Throat

Inflammation: When a physician looks at the ears, nose and throat, she or he is often looking for signs of infection and/or inflammation which will help point to the right diagnosis. Inflammation is a complex set of chemical reactions and changes that tissues undergo in response to bacterial invasion or other diseases. Tissues undergo this response to injury as an early attempt to prevent further injury, and as a means of beginning the healing process. The chemical reactions which occur act as signals which call different blood cells to the site of an injury. Some cells come to repair the damage while others come to fight the enemy (eg: a bacteria, virus, etc.).

There are many types of injuries which cause tissue inflammation including physical injuries (e.g. bruising and sprains, allergies and infections).

Infections occur when the tissues of the body are invaded by other living organisms which are not supposed to be living in that tissue. There are several types of organisms which can cause infections such as bacteria, viruses, parasites and fungi. When infection occurs in a tissue, there is almost always inflammation which accompanies it.

Doctors use four signs and symptoms to determine if inflammation may be present. The four hallmarks of inflammation are redness, pain, swelling and increased temperature. For example, if you were to fall and sprain your ankle, the body would respond to this injury with inflammation and your ankle would become swollen, tender, red looking and it would even feel hot to the touch.

When examining the ears, nose and throat, it is important to determine if any of these structures are inflamed. If they are, this is usually a sign of infection, but may be a sign of allergy or injury.

A. THE EARS:

Let us review some of the basics of the ear. The ear consists of three parts, the outer ear, the middle ear and the inner ear. **[Figure 4A]**

The outer ear: Only the outer ear is visible from the outside of the body. The outer ear is comprised of the unusually shaped pieces of cartilage (like soft bone) that appear on each side of the face, and includes the tube that leads all the way to the eardrum. The eardrum is a thin membrane that functions much like a sail on a boat. When sound waves (which are much like shifting wind, but on a microscopic scale) enter the ear they move the eardrum, much in the same way that wind moves the sails of a sailboat. This movement is then transferred to bones in the middle ear which in turn move and thus transmit the sound deeper into the ear.

The middle ear: The middle ear is a small, air-filled cavity directly behind the eardrum. At the back of this cavity is an area of spongy bone known as the mastoid. (The mastoid bone is located directly behind the ear, it's the part of your skull on which the tips of your glasses rest.)

The middle ear contains three small bones which connect the eardrum to the inner ear, and transmit the sound from the outer ear through the middle ear and into the inner ear where special nerves are located to decipher sound. The middle ear is connected to the back of the throat by a small collapsible tube, known as the eustachian tube. This tube allows air into the middle ear so that the pressure inside the middle equals that of the atmospheric pressure outside. This tube is especially important when travelling at high altitudes, or when diving deep below water. When pressures become unusually low or high it is important that the middle ear pressure equalize with the outside pressure. Sometimes infection in the nose or throat spreads through this tube into the middle ear causing it to become infected.

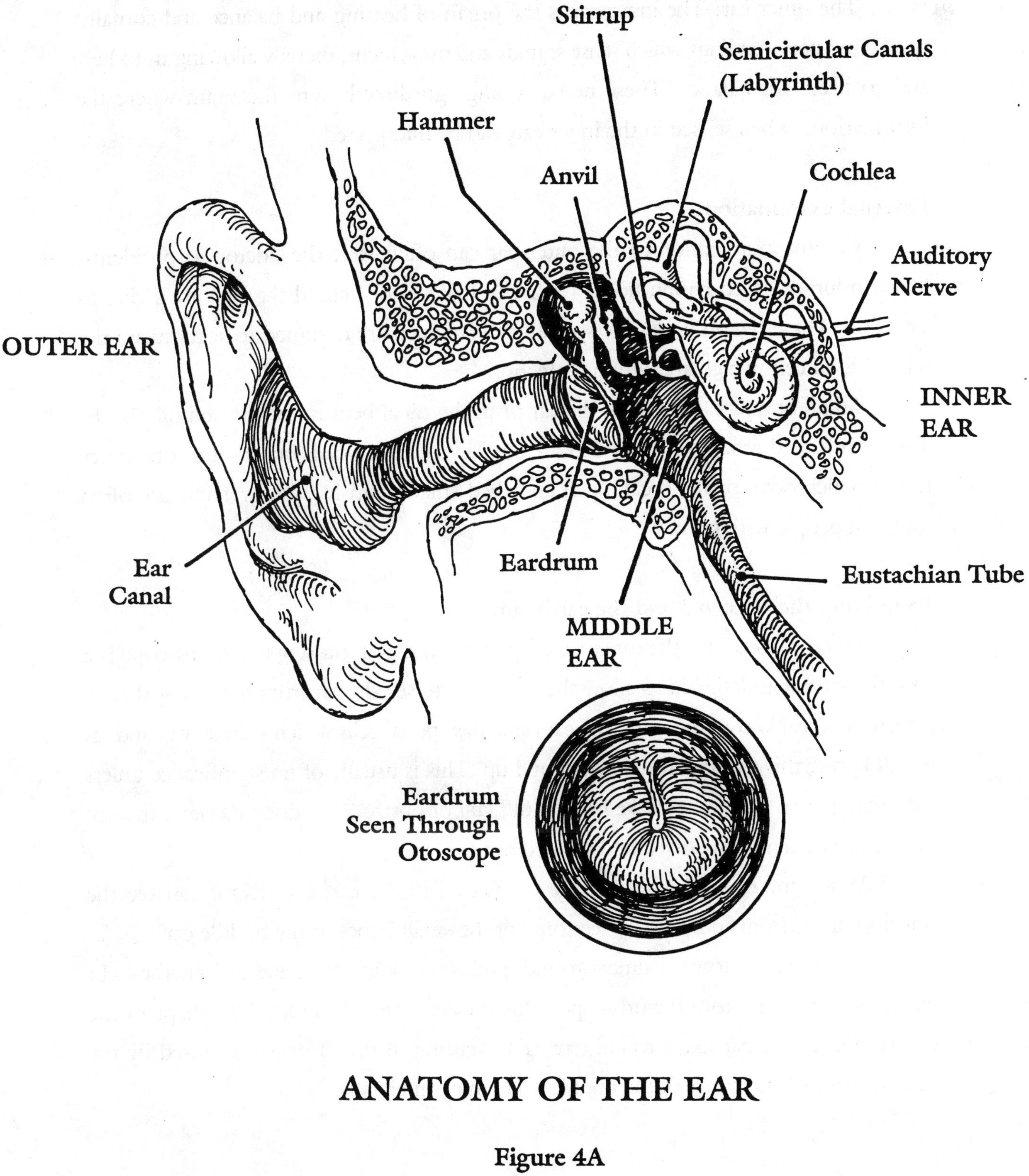

ANATOMY OF THE EAR

Figure 4A

The inner ear: The inner ear is the organ of hearing and balance and contains specialized nerve endings which sense sounds and movement, thereby allowing us to hear and to keep our balance. These nerve endings go directly into the brain where the information, when sensed in the inner ear, can be interpreted.

External examination:

Careful examination of the outer ear can often alert the doctor to problems. Swollen lumps called lymph nodes (either in front of or behind the ear) are a clue to infection. These lymph nodes are special glands which are designed to accumulate the white blood cells which are fighting infection.

Small bumps can form on the ear or in the canal because of blocked oil glands. These are called sebaceous cysts and are similar to acne. Small bumps are sometimes found which occasionally break open and shed small whitish crystals. These are often found in people with gout.

Examining the ear canal and the eardrum:

Doctors look into the ears of their patients using an otoscope. An otoscope is a special instrument designed to allow the physician to see the eardrum directly -- that is, if there is no ear wax in the way! The ear canal has special cells which secrete wax and, as we all know, this wax can sometimes build up. This is usually of no significance unless the buildup is so great as to make hearing difficult or obstruct the doctor's view. In such cases the wax can be dissolved and washed out.

When the otoscope is correctly positioned in the ear, the doctor can see the translucent eardrum and can also see some of the small bones in the middle ear.

A normal eardrum is almost round, pinkish-gray in color, and reflects the light which is coming in from the otoscope. This is called the light reflex. The shape of the eardrum is somewhat like a round tent. This tenting of the eardrum is caused by the malleus (one of the bones of the middle ear) which indents it.

In addition to looking at the ear, the physician can also observe the movement of the eardrum by pumping small amounts of air into the ear canal. Most otoscopes are designed to accept the attachment of a rubber tube with a bulb at the end (this attachment looks somewhat like an antique perfume bottle attachment). With the rubber tube and bulb attached, the physician can place the otoscope in the ear and blow air onto the eardrum. This is called pneumatic otoscopy. The normal ear drum will move in and out as the pressure increases and decreases. This is a sign that the middle ear is filled with air as it should be.

Some diseases diagnosed by examining the ear:

When the outer ear and ear canal become infected, they exhibit the typical signs and symptoms of inflammation and become red, warm, swollen and tender. This diagnosis can be easily made because it is painful to pull on the cartilage of the outer ear and the ear canal looks red and swollen. Doctors call infection of the outer ear *otitis externa*. A common example of this would be the infection which people call swimmer's ear.

When the middle ear becomes infected it too becomes inflamed, but since the physician cannot see directly into it (the eardrum obscures this view), other signs and symptoms must be relied upon. In middle ear infection the eardrum becomes red and the normal light reflected off the eardrum makes it appear dull and less transparent. Small blood vessels in the eardrum appear which are barely visible. Also, fluid or pus may collect behind the eardrum and this can sometimes be seen with the otoscope. If fluid cannot be seen, and the doctor still suspects infection, she or he may choose to do pneumatic otoscopy to see if the eardrum moves freely. Fluid behind the eardrum causes it to move slowly, or not at all. Sometimes fluid or pus will collect under such pressure that it causes the eardrum to burst. The doctor may see pus (yellow colored fluid) in the outer ear canal. When the middle ear is infected, otitis media is diagnosed and antibiotic therapy is usually required because the infection is often caused by bacteria. The patient may even have an earache and fever, which are additional signs of infection.

The mastoid bone and its small air chambers sometimes become infected also, and this is called mastoiditis. Here the bone behind the ear is tender, and there may be redness and swelling.

Occasionally there may be fluid behind the eardrum which is not pus. Such a fluid is called an effusion and can be due to a viral infection or to the trauma caused by changing pressures. Antibiotics are not utilized since viruses do not respond to antibiotic treatment. Fever and pain can always be treated, but the viral infection must be left to run its course.

Rarely, the outer ear can become painful and have blisters in the canal and on the eardrum. This infection is caused by a virus as well. There is frequently an earache associated with this condition and the fluid which drains may even have blood in it.

Tests for hearing:

The standard physical examination does not usually include tests for hearing since patients often report if there is a hearing problem. Tests of hearing are more important in children who are less able to explain that they are not able to hear well. A child who has had a serious ear infection can have some hearing loss for several months after the infection has ended, and testing is sometimes warranted. Children should have one formal hearing test before entering school, and they should be tested immediately if their speech is delayed. Poor hearing is often a cause of delayed speech development in children.

Two types of hearing loss:

There are two different types of hearing loss and each has different causes. The first is hearing loss due to problems with conducting sound through the outer and middle ear and into the inner ear where the specialized nerve endings are located. Causes include: wax in the ear, hardening of the bones of the middle ear, fluid in the middle ear and a hole in the eardrum. This type of hearing loss is called conductive loss and is the most common type in people below the age of 40. The second type of hearing loss occurs when the sensory cells (which are designed to collect the sound) and nerves are not transmitting sound effectively to the brain, or when the brain has difficulty receiving them. Causes include: aging deafness, drug-induced nerve damage to the nerves of hearing, and excessive exposure to loud noise. This type of hearing loss is called sensorineural loss and is most common in adults over the age of 40.

There are two simple tests to help distinguish these two types of hearing loss: Rinne's Test and Weber's Test. Each is conducted with the use of a tuning fork which can be struck, causing it to vibrate at a certain frequency.

Weber Test: The doctor strikes the tuning fork and places the base of it in the middle of the patient's head at the top, asking in which ear the sound is the loudest. Normally, the sound is equal in both ears. If the noise is heard louder in one ear, this is abnormal. If an ear has sensorineural loss, the sound will seem softer in that ear. [Figure 4B]

Rinne Test: The doctor strikes the tuning fork and places its base against the mastoid bone of the patient's ear (behind the ear). The patient is told to inform the doctor when sound is no longer heard. This is the time when bone conduction of sound stops. At this point, the doctor moves the vibrating ends of the tuning fork to within 1-2 inches of the patient's ear and asks if the sound can be heard again. The answer should be yes, since air conduction is normally better (louder and longer) than bone conduction. If a patient has conduction hearing loss, the sound will be heard louder and longer while the tuning fork is against the bone than when the sound is only traveling through air. This is a negative Rinne test and it is abnormal. A positive Rinne test (normal) is when the sound is heard longer through the air.

The hearing of babies can be crudely tested by making a sound near the baby's ear (such as snapping the fingers), and seeing if her or his eyes blink. This is called the acoustic blink reflex.

Other tests:

Audiometry: When hearing loss is strongly suspected or documented by Rinne's and Weber's tests, more sophisticated tests of hearing can be done. Patients can be tested

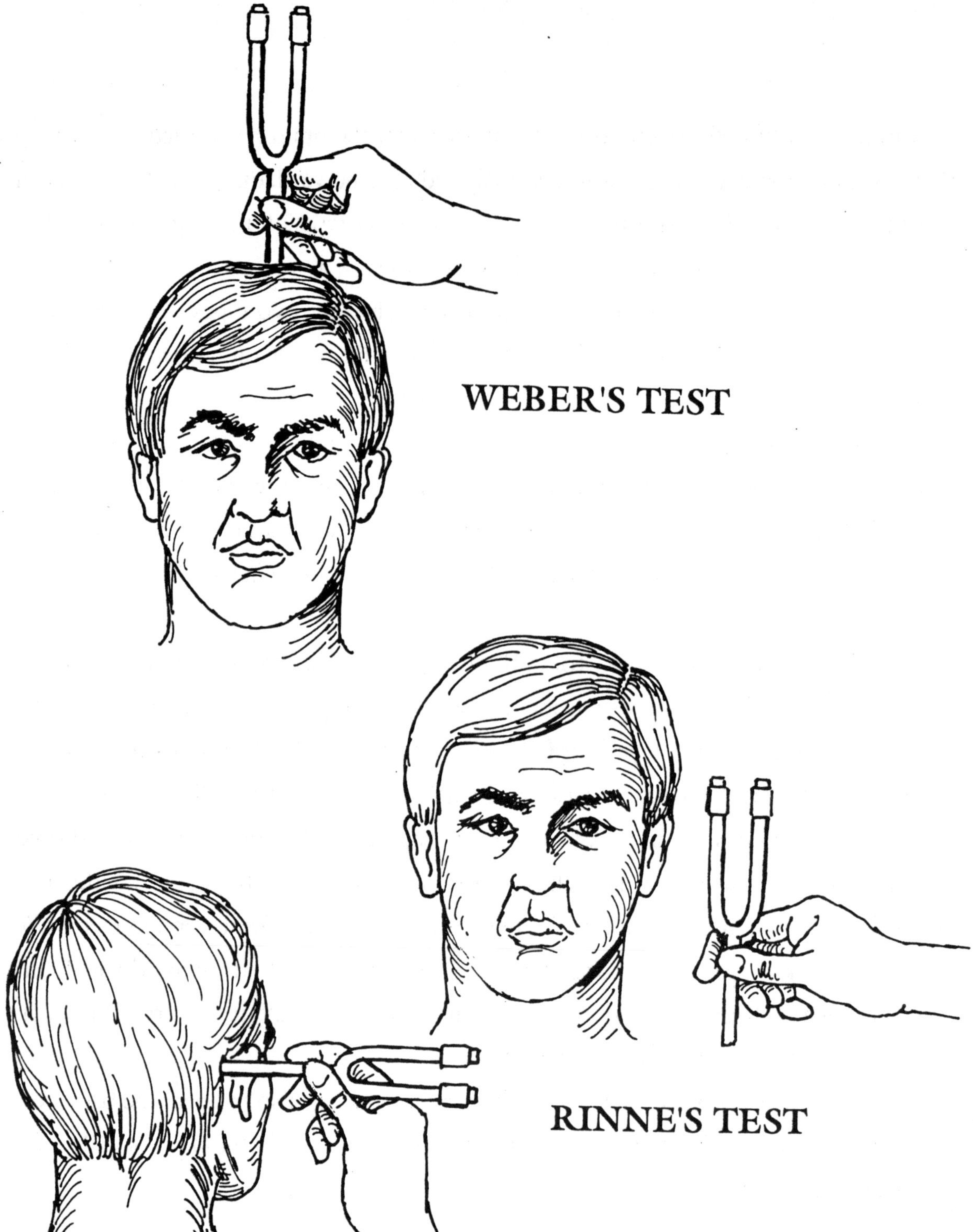

HEARING TESTS

Figure 4B

at different frequencies and volumes with audiometric equipment to determine exactly the amount of loss.

B. THE NOSE:

Upper respiratory infections are among the most common human ailments. They often start in the nose and throat, but frequently affect the ears and lungs. Most upper respiratory infections are caused by viruses, however, some are due to bacteria.

A complete physical examination should include a careful examination of the nose, especially in someone with symptoms of an upper respiratory infection -- such as cough, sore throat, "runny nose", and fever. The physician can look into the nose with a special attachment which fits onto the otoscope and can see the mucous membranes in the nose. The doctor should see a moist, pinkish surface. Sometimes the membrane is more red than normal and has a lot of clear fluid coming out of it. This points to viral infection. Sometimes the membrane is more red than normal and has a lot of yellowish or brownish fluid coming out of it. This points to bacterial infection. The membrane can appear pale or whitish in color and be covered with a clear fluid, and this usually indicates that the symptoms are due to an allergy instead of infection. In addition to color changes, several other observations help to make a diagnosis. Polyps are outgrowths of the membrane which occur often in people with allergies such as "hay fever". Bleeding spots indicate areas which have been inflamed for so long that the irritation has caused a break in the membrane. Examining the nose can help the doctor to see objects that children may have placed in their noses. Areas that are pre-cancerous can often be removed before they become dangerous.

C. SINUSES:

After examining the nose, the doctor may choose to tap on the head over the sinuses to see if they are infected. Recall that infected tissue is tender. So if one taps over the maxillary sinus (over the cheek bone) or over the frontal sinuses (over the eyebrow), this may cause sharp pain which indicates that the patient may have a sinus infection. The doctor may shine a light into the sinuses through the skin and see if the light passes through. An infected and clogged up sinus will usually not allow light to pass through it. You can try this on your own by getting in a dark room and pressing a small flashlight onto your cheek (just below your eye). You should be able to see the light shining through and glowing inside your mouth!

D. NECK PALPATION:

A physician may also examine a patient's neck for additional clues to make a diagnosis. Again, this examination usually begins with inspection. An enlarged area of the neck may indicate a thyroid disorder (in which case the mass may be called a goiter). The doctor then begins systematically palpating the neck to identify any abnormalities. Many times lymph nodes will be felt which may indicate infection. Palpable lymph nodes, however, may also be present in healthy individuals.

E. THE MOUTH AND THROAT:

So why does my doctor say, "open your mouth and say 'Ah'?" This is to get a better look at the back of the throat. When we say "Ah", our tongue is pressed into the bottom of the mouth and the doctor can see better. If the patient doesn't open wide enough, or the tongue is not on the bottom of the mouth, the doctor may place a tongue depressor in the mouth and press the tongue down.

It is important to examine the mouth, because abnormalities can be helpful in diagnosing diseases in their early stages. In examining the mouth the doctor usually looks in with a light and then can feel areas of abnormality with his or her fingers. The tongue, teeth, gums, roof and floor of the mouth should be inspected first, and then later the physician can look at the tonsils and throat. A sore in the mouth could be as simple as a canker sore, but it could also be a cold sore from herpes infection or the chancre sore of early syphilis. Small areas of red or whitish discoloration could point to early cancer, and it is especially important to look for them in patients who use any tobacco products. Sometimes the inside of the mouth can become coated with white spots, and this may indicate infection with a fungus called Candida. Most people know this infection as thrush, and it is commonly seen in infants.

The tonsils and throat are usually examined to look for infection. Since the tonsil is just a specialized lymph node, it frequently swells and becomes tender when infection is present. When the tonsils are infected they look like bright red olives, speckled with yellow pus spots. When a doctor sees these, it is likely that one of two infections is present: "strep throat" or mononucleosis. Both of these infections can be serious and need medical treatment.

Finally, the back of the throat is examined. It, too, is a mucous membrane and shows the same signs of infection as other membranes which we have discussed. When inflamed it becomes tender, red and swollen. These signs, in combination with fever, usually indicate infection of the throat.

Appearance of the throat in different infections:

Viral infection -- redness, prominent bumps on the back of the throat which are swelling of lymph tissue.

Mononucleosis (Epstein Bar Virus) -- red dots on the roof of the mouth, enlarged lymph nodes around the ears, and in the neck.

Strep throat -- Swollen tonsils, yellow patches on the tonsils, swollen and tender lymph nodes in the neck.

Diphtheria (now very rare due to immunization) -- dull red color of the throat with a thick gray layer of fluid.

Most infection is caused by viruses, but since those caused by bacteria can be serious if left untreated, most doctors will choose to culture the throat when infection is diagnosed. A culture is made by swabbing the throat with a cotton tip and transferring the bacteria onto a special jelly plate which is put in an incubator and allowed to grow. Laboratory technologists are able to determine exactly which bacteria is causing the infection, and let the doctor know which antibiotic will best treat the infection. Throat cultures are expensive and time-consuming, so some doctors choose to do a quick test in the office. This way, immediate treatment can begin without waiting for the bacteria to grow. This quick test involves placing a swab into the back of the throat to obtain some fluid. This fluid is then mixed with chemical reagents. The type of chemical reaction observed indicates the presence of certain kinds of bacteria.

F. OTHER TESTS:

Patients with complaints such as hoarseness or difficulty swallowing need more extensive evaluations of their mouths and throats and these cannot be performed with the usual equipment. There are special instruments which enable the doctor to see down into the throat and into the back of the nose, but these are reserved for special cases and are not included in the routine physical examination.

G. THE IMPORTANCE OF TREATING STREP THROAT:

Each year, many people are treated for strep throat, a fairly common ailment. People with strep throat usually have a sore throat and fever. The usual treatment is 10 days of Penicillin. Most patients don't know why their doctor want them to take medicine for 10 days when they usually feel better after three or four days. The reason has nothing to do with the sore throat or how the patient feels, but relates to the fact that if strep throat is not treated completely, it can lead to rheumatic fever, which can destroy the valves of the heart. The most common reason (worldwide) for trouble with heart valves is rheumatic fever from a sore throat, which was caused by strep, and was not treated with a full 10 days of Penicillin! So if your doctor diagnoses strep throat, be sure to take the full 10 days of treatment, even if your throat feels better long before 10 days.

CHAPTER 5

The Eyes

Examination of the eyes is always an important part of the physical examination. In addition to detecting the diseases which affect the eyes directly, a doctor can see things in examining the eyes which are signs of the overall health of the body. For example, the eyes can be used to follow the course of such common and potentially dangerous diseases as diabetes and high blood pressure.

First, review the diagram **(Figure 5A)** of the eye and learn some of the structures which will be discussed below.

A. The Outside of the Eyes:

The first part of a careful eye examination is inspection of the structures which surround the eye, such as the eyebrows, eyelids, eyelashes and even the holes in the skull (called the orbits) which surround and protect the eye. For the most part, everyone knows what normal eyes look like, but in illness there can be subtle changes which indicate the presence of disease.

There are a number of conditions affecting the appearance of the outer eye:

1)"Black eye" occurs when the soft tissues around the eye, such as the upper and lower eyelid are damaged. Small vessels in these tissues are broken and bleed, causing a brown appearance around the eye.

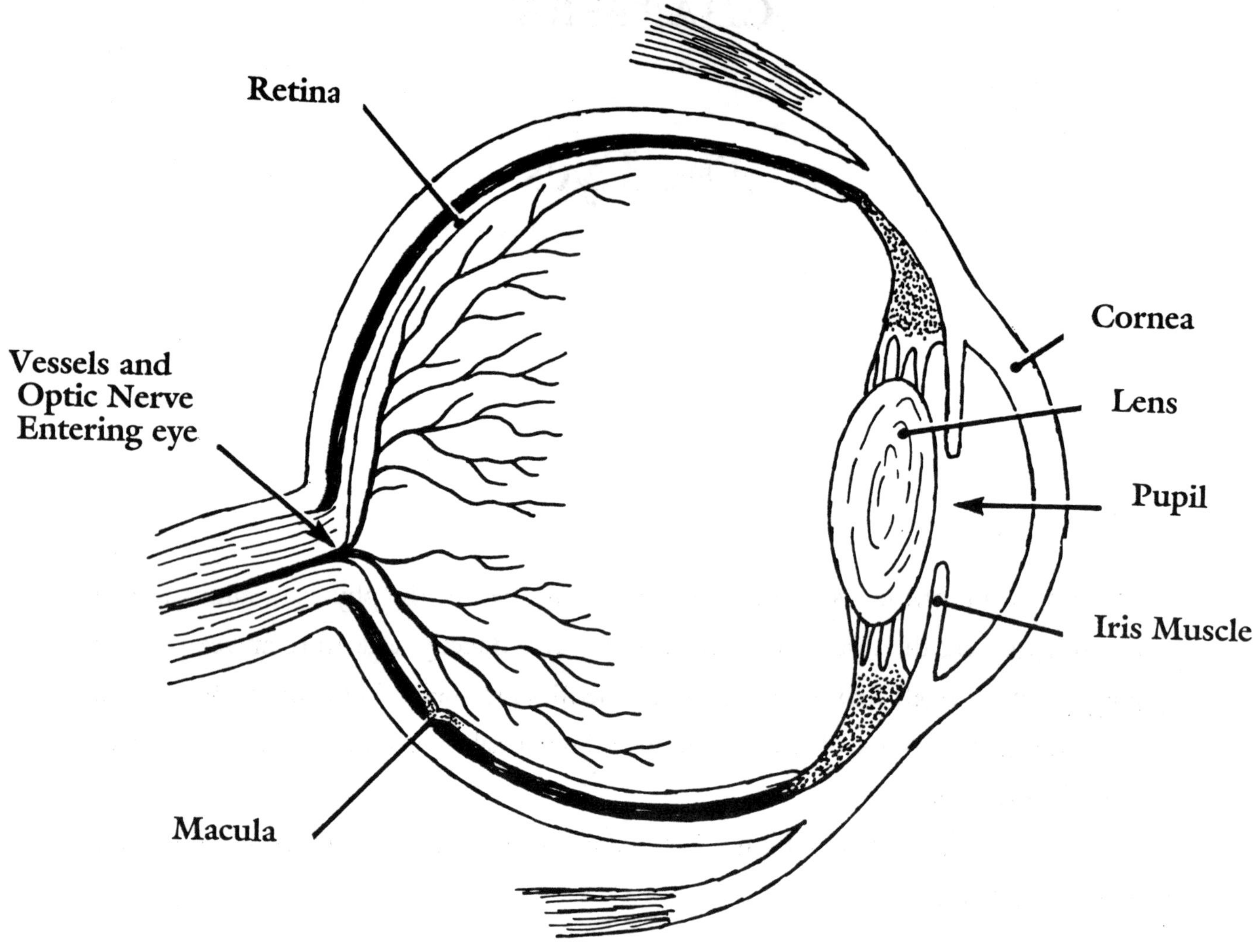

ANATOMY OF THE EYE

Figure 5A

2) Sometimes the tiny lining (membrane) which surrounds the eye and protects it can become damaged, and it too can bleed. In this situation, the blood collects between this lining (called the conjunctiva) and the hard white eyeball (called the sclera) and it looks like a red puddle in the white of the eye. Doctors call this sub-conjunctival hemorrhage, because it is bleeding which occurs below the conjunctiva.

3) When the liver fails to function correctly and get rid of all of the bile which is produced there daily, the whites of the eyes may become yellow/green in appearance, indicating that there is some disease affecting the liver or gall bladder. Some people call this "yellow jaundice". Bile, by the way, is used by the body to help digest fats in the diet.

4) "Pink eye" occurs when bacteria or viruses invade and infect the hair follicles on the eyelid. Local inflammation occurs, causing pain, swelling, redness and increased temperature of these tissues.

5) People who have hyperthyroidism (too much of the hormone that speeds up the body's metabolic rate) often have eyes which protrude. Their eyes actually bulge out, making them look as if they are trying to hold their eyes open as wide as possible.

6)In addition to looking at the eyes, there are times when it is helpful to feel the eyes, and their sockets in order to detect problems. Anyone who has been in an accident, for instance, should have a careful examination of their eye sockets to see if there is any tenderness which could mean a fracture of their skull.

7) People with complaints of dry or teary eyes should have the tearing system of their eyes examined. There are glands in the upper outer lid above each eye which secrete tears to lubricate the eye's outer lining (conjunctiva). The tears, in the form of a fine layer of fluid, bathe the eye as they flow downward and inward to collecting sacs which are located at the inner lower part of the eyelid of each eye. (Gently pull your lower eyelid down in front of a mirror and see if you can see the small hole where your tears drain.) From there tears drain into the nose, which is why your nose runs when you cry -- when extra tears are draining! To examine whether or not this conducting

system is infected, the doctor can press on the sac (located in the lower eyelid nearest the nose) and see that only clear fluid comes out, not colored fluid or pus.

B. The Movements of the Eyes:

There are several ways in which the eyes move, and each can be compared to the operation of a camera. First, the eyeballs themselves move in order to allow people to look at different things without having to move their heads. This is like moving a camera in order to point at the subject being photographed. Second, the pupils get larger and smaller in order to control the amount of light which enters the back part of the eye. This is similar to the movement of the aperture in the lens of the camera. Finally, the muscles which surround the lens of the eye move, thereby changing the shape of the lens. This allows the person to focus on objects which are at different distances from the eye. In a similar way, the lens of a camera can be manually moved to focus on objects at different distances from the camera.

The movements of each eyeball are controlled by six muscles, which are precisely controlled by special nerves which exit the brain. The movement of the eyes should be tested during the physical examination. The eyes must move in perfect synchrony or the person will see double. This function of the eyes has more to do with the brain than the eye itself, since nerves coming from the brain control the muscles that coordinate these intricate movements.

The eyes are not only designed to move together in complete coordination with each other, but are also designed to move in coordination with the body's movements so that objects can be kept in focus at all times, even when moving. If your eyes were not coordinated in this way, when you walked, everything would be blurred by your movements! When we move, our inner ear senses this movement and tells our brain exactly what type of movement is occurring. The brain then signals the muscles of the eye to move the eyes in such a way as to keep everything that we see in the same place in our visual field, so that it does not appear blurred. You have no doubt heard of hand-eye coordination -- well, this is ear-eye coordination, and it is much more accurate than hand-eye coordination!

You can illustrate how this works by doing a simple experiment. Hold your hand twelve inches in front of your face and move it back and forth rapidly. Your eyes will not be able to keep up with the movements of your hand and it will appear blurred (That's as good as your hand-eye coordination gets!). Now hold your hand in the same place, and this time move your head side to side rapidly. This time you will notice that you are able to focus on the same place of your hand, and that nothing is blurred. Your inner ear is telling your brain the exact movements of your head, and your brain is then sending the eye signals about how to correct their positions so as to keep everything in sharp focus. Amazing!

A doctor inspecting the eyes will always make sure that the pupils are of equal size and that they react briskly to different intensities of light. This test is easily done by shining a penlight into one eye and watching for the opposite pupil to get smaller. If a person has pupils which are of different sizes it could mean that some part of their nervous system is not functioning properly. If their pupils are very large and do not constrict in response to light, this could indicate brain damage or coma, and if their pupils are very small it could indicate that they have overdosed on certain drugs or medications.

The muscles which change the shape of the lens allow a person to focus on near and far objects at different times. These muscles are rarely involved in diseases, but can sometimes be involved when people have blurred vision and need corrective lenses.

C. The Function of the Eyes:

Since the function of the eyes is to see objects both far and near, and since we all rely heavily on our sense of sight, any physical examination should always include a test of one's ability to see. The best way to do this test (called a test of visual acuity) is to have someone attempt to read a wall chart at a distance of 20 feet. Each eye is tested separately. In some settings where a wall chart is not available or where there are not 20 feet of space available, a person can be asked to read some small news print of differing sizes to get a crude estimate of the sharpness of their eyesight.

In addition to testing visual acuity it is important to test how well a person can see with their peripheral vision, that is, how well they see the things to either side of them which are not directly in their line of sight. If you are watching television and someone walks into the room to your left or right side you are aware of their presence and motion, even though you are not looking directly at them. This function of your eyes, called peripheral vision, is extremely important. It is important to test this vision because some people can have marked loss in their peripheral vision in advanced diseases of the eye, or other systemic diseases, without even knowing it. Peripheral vision is usually tested by a doctor having you look directly at her or his nose while placing a number of fingers at various positions in your peripheral vision and asking you to count the number of fingers that you see. This is a crude method of testing. Precise testing can be completed by an ophthamologist (eye specialist in medicine) on anyone who demonstrates a deficiency, or has a disease which merits careful and precise peripheral field monitoring.

D. The Inside of the Eye:

It is important to inspect the inside of the eye for two reasons. First, the retina (lining in the back of the eyeball) is the only place in the body where one can see small arteries, veins and nerves directly. Second, the things which can be seen by a simple eye examination are often important clues to other diseases which affect the whole body, such as high blood pressure and diabetes.

The eye is inspected with the aid of a special light called an ophthalmoscope. **[Figure 5B]** It is a light with several lenses which allow the doctor to see through the pupil and into the back of the eye where the retina is located. First, the room is darkened to allow the patient's pupils to enlarge so that more can be seen. (If this amount of darkness is not sufficient to allow the pupil to be seen clearly, then special eye drops are placed in the eye to dilate the pupil.) The doctor then asks the patient to

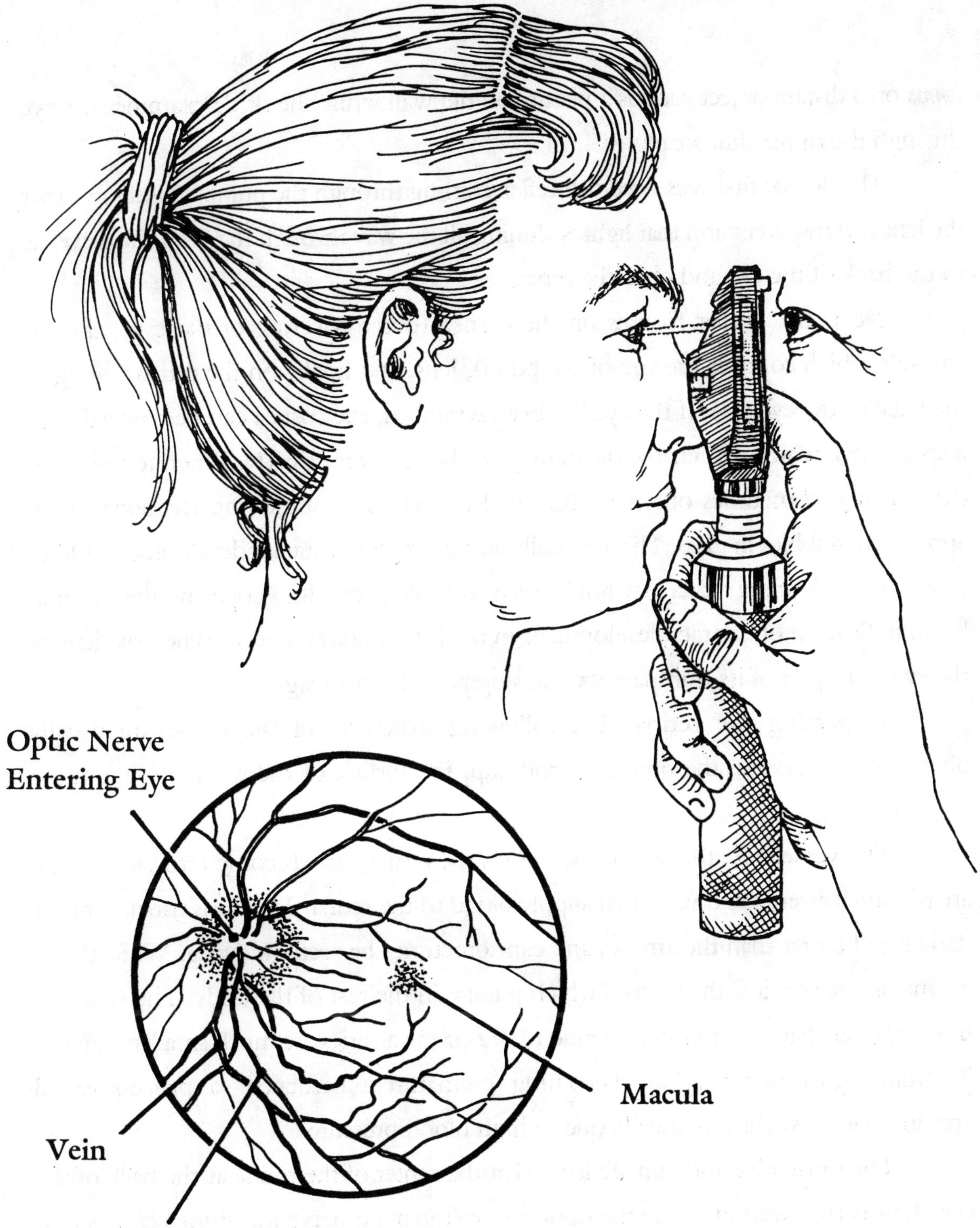

THE OPHTHALMOSCOPE

Figure 5B

focus on a distant object such as a picture on the wall while she or he examines the eye through the ophthalmoscope.

The doctor first sees a reddish reflex coming through the pupil. This shows that the lens is transparent and that light is shining all the way through the fluid-filled eyeball to the back of the eye and onto the retina.

Next, the doctor focuses on the cornea (outer covering of the eye), the iris (muscle which controls the size of the pupil), lens, and finally on the retina (lining in the back of the eyeball). If the eye has been scratched, the cornea can be covered with a special dye which will enable the damage to be seen very clearly. When focusing on the lens it is sometimes observed that the lens may have some imperfections which appear like bubbles in glass. This is usually an early sign of cataract development. Other times, the back of the retina may not be seen with the ophthalmoscope and this too may be an indication of cataract development in the lens. Cataracts occur when the lens of the eye loses part of its transparency, causing partial loss of sight.

Inspecting the retina: The following structures of the retina are usually observed: the vessels, the optic disc and cup, the surface of the retina itself and the macula.

The vessels: As the doctor focuses on the retina, vessels come into view which are the small arteries and veins that supply blood to the retina. The veins usually appear darker and larger than the arteries and can sometimes be seen pulsating. While this is normal in the eye, it is the arteries which pulsate in the rest of the body. The veins are usually larger than the arteries by a ratio of 3:2. If the arteries are much smaller than this it could signal that they are becoming prematurely hardened (a process called arteriolosclerosis which is usually due to high blood pressure).

The optic disc and cup are located at the center of the retina at the back of the eye. This is the location where the optic nerve (the main nerve for vision) comes into the back of the eyeball. It is here that nerves can be seen directly. The disc appears as a circle of reddish-brown color, while the cup is a smaller circle inside the disc which is more yellowish and pink in color.

The cup is the head of the optic nerve. Normally, the cup and disc are round and have distinct, clear margins or edges. The cup should have a diameter less than, or equal to, one third the diameter of the disc. Sometimes the cup may be enlarged beyond this normal amount. This can signal that glaucoma is present.

Glaucoma is a disease of the eye in which pressure builds up in the eyeball, which can eventually cause blindness. This disease often occurs without symptoms, so people don't know that anything is wrong. It is easily diagnosed and treated and since it is a preventable cause of blindness, it is a good reason to have a regular eye exam. An ophthamologist or optometrist can quickly test the pressure in the eye by blowing a puff of air onto the eye. A machine calculates the pressure in the eye based on the resistance that the puff of air encounters. High pressure indicates glaucoma.

The surface of the retina is reddish brown in color and has blood vessels coursing all through it, much like a cobweb spread over a flat surface. Vessels leaking blood or other fluid onto the retina indicate that something is wrong.

The macula is an area at the midline of the retina. To see this area, the doctor asks the patient to look directly into the light coming from the ophthalmoscope. The macula of the retina is usually more dusky appearing and has no vessels crossing it.

Vessels: the condition of the vessels of the retina can serve as indicators of certain diseases. If these vessels are unusually small, for example, this could indicate high blood pressure. If they are more numerous than usual and appear to be forming even more new vessels, this can be a sign that a person has diabetes or that their diabetes is poorly controlled. Sometimes the vessels can break and blood is lost onto the surface of the retina. This can be seen in such diseases as high blood pressure, diabetes, leukemia and also in individuals with severe bleeding disorders.

A POSSIBLE EMERGENCY -- INCREASED PRESSURE IN THE BRAIN:

Finally, the eye exam can be used as a means of determining something about the pressure in the fluid surrounding the brain. (It is important to know something about the pressure in the brain since abnormally high pressure has many causes, but is almost always dangerous and needs urgent attention.) Since the optic nerve comes into the back of the eye, and since it is surrounded by the fluid which surrounds the brain, changes in the eye can be seen when the pressure of this fluid becomes too high. When the pressure in the fluid surrounding the brain becomes abnormally high, the optic nerve swells and the borders blur (this is called papilledema). As this swelling increases, the veins in the retina often stop their usual pulsating and the optic cup enlarges and bulges into the back of the eye. This can often be seen through the ophthalmoscope.

CHAPTER 6

The Heart and Circulation

We all know that the heart pumps blood to the rest of the body and that without a healthy heart, none of us would survive. In fact, about 50% of the people living in an industrialized society will eventually die from diseases related to the heart and circulation. Most of these conditions are avoidable by eating properly, exercising regularly, stopping smoking and drinking alcohol only in moderation. But how exactly does a physician examine the heart and know whether or not it is functioning properly?

A complete evaluation of the heart and its function includes taking a detailed history, doing a physical examination, taking a chest x-ray and doing an electrocardiogram. There are several other tests which could also be done, but these are usually reserved for people with specific symptoms and signs which indicate the possibility of heart disease.

The goal of examining the heart is not only to determine if there is any disease, but to decide whether the problem is in the small vessels which actually supply blood to the muscle of the heart (coronary arteries are like three straws lying on the surface and penetrating the muscular walls of the heart itself) or in the valves (the doors between the rooms or chambers of the heart). Further, one needs to determine whether the problem is on the left or right side of the heart. The left side of the heart pumps blood to most of the body under high pressure (which we measure as blood pressure). The right side of the heart receives blood from all over the body and pumps it to the lungs to be oxygenated before it is returned to the heart. This side operates under low pressure. **[Figure 6A]** Also, problems could relate to the internal nervous system of the heart which coordinates its pumping action.

A. The History: The following symptoms are generally considered to be important in assessing heart functioning: shortness of breath, swelling of ankles (edema), feeling one's own heart beating fast (palpitations), dizziness or fainting (syncope), and chest pain. These symptoms should be reported whenever they occur.

Some symptoms occur primarily with left-sided heart disease, while others occur predominantly with right-sided heart disease. For example, swelling of the legs and a swollen liver and abdomen usually suggests right-sided heart disease. Shortness of breath and fatigue usually suggest left-sided heart disease.

B. The Physical Examination: The only special equipment needed for this examination is the stethoscope and a penlight.

1. Looking (Inspection): The first thing that a physician will do in examining the heart is to observe the patient and look for signs of heart disease. The skin should be carefully examined to look for discoloration (blueness) which could indicate that the tissues are not receiving enough oxygenated blood. The skin can also show signs of too much cholesterol in the blood (which is dangerous for the heart). For example, some people with high cholesterol will have deposits of cholesterol under their skin which appear as little lumps (or nodules) on the elbows or on the eyelids. Others with abnormally high cholesterol levels may have rings of whitish-yellow cholesterol deposits around the edge of their eyes (this is called arcus senilis and is considered normal in people over the age of 60). The fingernails are examined for rounded nails (called clubbing) which indicate long term (or chronic) lack of oxygen. This can be seen in many smokers with emphysema. The patient should also be observed for swelling of the ankles

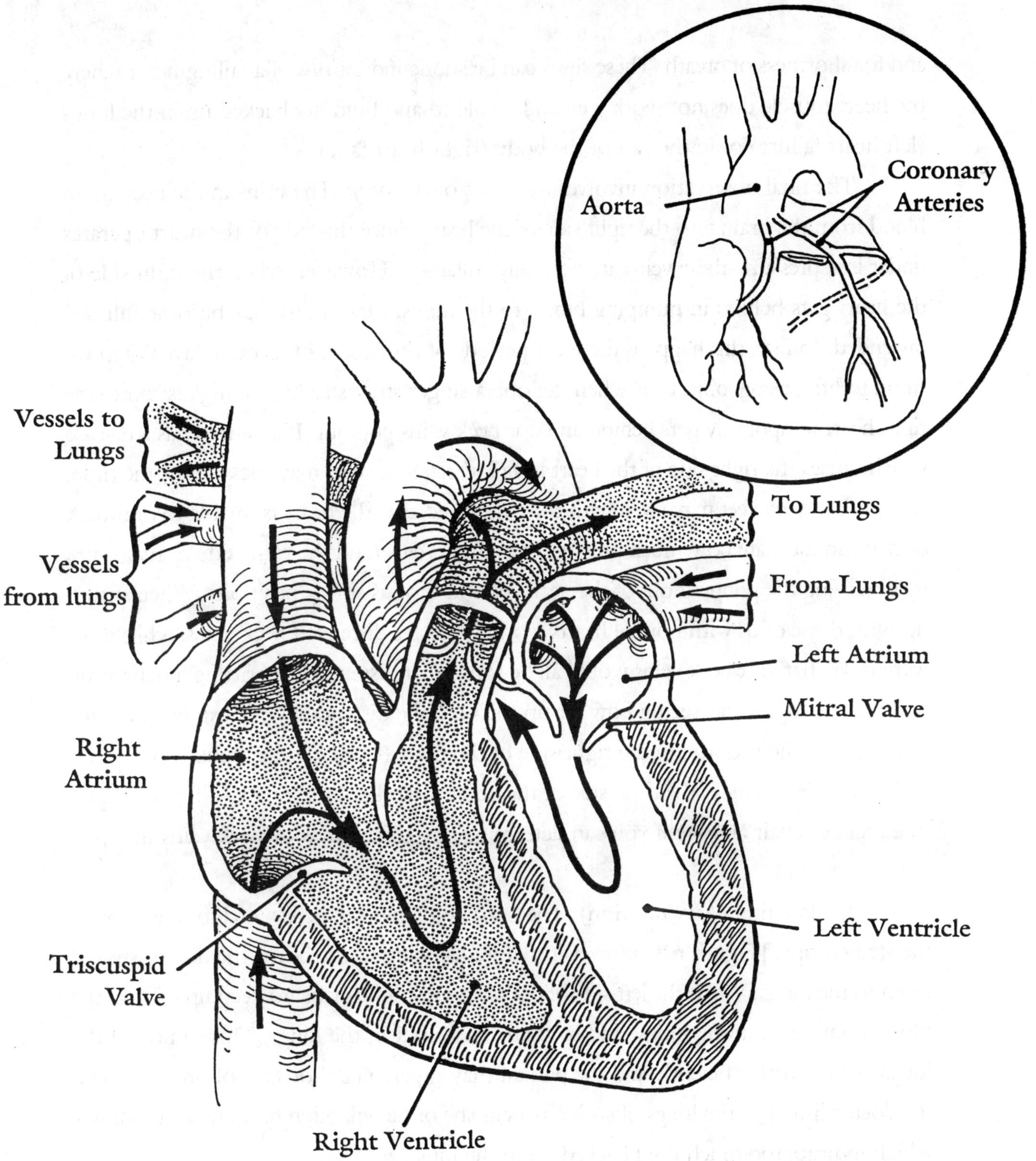

ANATOMY OF THE HEART

Figure 6A

and for shortness of breath. These signs can be subtle indications of a failing heart where the heart muscle does not work well and so blood and fluid get backed up in the lungs (left heart failure) or in the rest of the body (right heart failure).

The final observation involves the veins of the neck. The veins in the neck drain blood from the brain into the right side of the heart. Since this side of the heart operates under low pressure, these veins are normally collapsed. However, when the right side of the heart gets behind in pumping blood to the lungs, these veins may become full and distended. In fact, this happens for short periods of time to all of us each day. When we strain to lift a heavy object, or when the opera singer strains to hit the highest note, the right heart temporarily gets behind and our neck veins pop out. If a patient has a disease which causes the right side of the heart to fail, their neck veins may stick out all the time. In addition, their feet may swell with the extra fluid that the heart is unable to pump. A doctor can estimate how much pressure is in these veins (and the right side of the heart) by observing the popping out of the neck veins in various sitting positions. When sitting upright, those of us with normal hearts would not have distended neck veins, while if we were to lay flat, our neck veins would all be somewhat distended. By sitting a patient up at different angles and seeing how far up the neck the distended veins extend, a doctor can estimate the pressure in the right side of the heart (called jugular venous pressure), and hence, determine if the right side of the heart is weak. Try sitting at different angles in a recliner chair and see if you can determine at what angle your neck veins first pop out.

2. Listening (Auscultation): The heart and lungs can be listened to directly with the stethoscope. **[Figure 6B]** However, before listening to the heart, the doctor should listen to the lungs. When the left side of the heart fails, it is unable to keep up with all the blood coming from the lungs, and so fluid can collect in the lungs. This can cause the lungs not to work efficiently and the patient may experience shortness of breath. When the doctor listens to the lungs of such a patient she or he will often hear crackling sounds which indicate too much fluid backed up in the lungs.

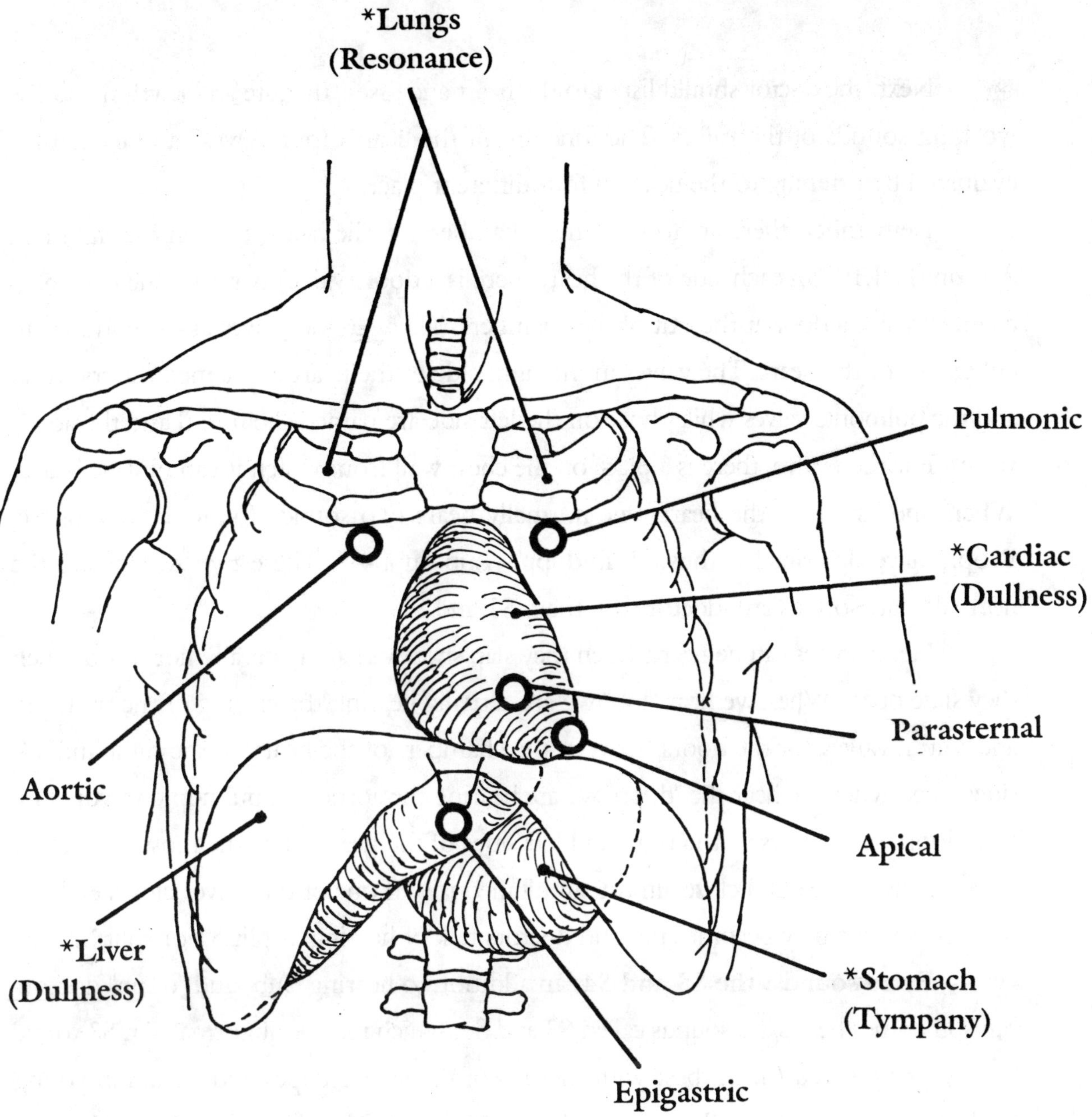

Five listening areas of the heart (without *)
Sounds heard with percussion of these areas of the various organs (with *)

AUSCULTATION OF HEART AND LUNGS

Figure 6B

Next, the doctor should listen to the heart and assess the rate and rhythm and the working sounds of the valves. The function of the heart's four valves can be carefully evaluated by listening to the heart in four different places.

Remember, there are four rooms (chambers) in the heart, two on the right and two on the left. On each side of the heart there is a door (valve) between the two main chambers and a door at the exit of the chambers. There are no valves at the entrance to either side of the heart. The valves in the right side of the heart are named the tricuspid and the pulmonic valves while those on the left side are named the mitral and the aortic valves. For each valve, there is a place on the chest wall from which it can best be heard. When one listens to the heart, one normally hears two sounds followed by a pause. People have described it thus: "Lub-dupp---Lub-dupp---". These two sounds are the normal heart sounds and doctors call them S1 and S2.

Heart valves can be heard when they slap shut, and are generally not heard when they slide open. When we hear "lub" we are actually hearing the closing of the tricuspid and mitral valves (or the doors between the chambers of the heart on the right and left sides), and when we hear the "dupp" we are hearing the aortic and pulmonic valves close (the doors at the exits to the right and left sides of the heart). For the most part, these pairs of valves open and close almost simultaneously. If one of the valves closes early or late, the sounds may become split and doctors talk of hearing a split S1 or split S2.

Extra sounds: the S3 and S4: In addition to hearing "lub" and "dupp" doctors can sometimes hear extra sounds called S3 and S4, which may be abnormal. An S3 sound is very low pitched (heard best with the bell of the stethoscope) and occurs in young adults and when there is a fluid overload on either side of the heart. An S4 sound is also very low pitched and occurs when the left or right ventricle is stiff and resistant to the flow to incoming blood.

Murmurs: A murmur is what a doctor hears when the valves of the heart are stuck and don't open or close all the way. There are three causes of murmurs. The first is caused by a leaking valve which allows blood to escape backwards and through it. This process is called regurgitation. The second type of murmur is caused by the damage or scarring of a valve. When this occurs the valve narrows, and the blood passes through the valve when it is only half open. Thus, the sound of blood rushing through the narrowed opening makes a humming sound. This narrowing is called a stenosis. The third type of murmur is caused by a hole in the wall between two of the heart's chambers. The blood leaking through this opening produces a sound recognizable as a murmur. Physicians are able to determine what kind of murmur a patient has by when in the pumping cycle it occurs, how long it lasts, what its pitch is, whether or not its sound tapers and, if so, by how much, how loud it is, from which listening position it is loudest, which activities make it louder or softer, and whether or not it radiates and can be heard in other areas. A few murmurs are normal, especially in children who have a lot of blood flowing around very fast in a very small space.

In addition to normal heart sounds and murmurs, there are at least three other sounds which can be heard: the rub, the click, and the snap.

Rub: The heart is surrounded by a sac which is filled with a small amount of fluid enabling it to slide freely as it moves while pumping. In some diseases, this sac may become inflamed, or become filled with large amounts of fluid. When this happens, the heart does not move freely in its protective sac and its movement has a scratching sound -- almost like opening velcro -- this sound is called a rub.

Clicks: Clicks are heard in the pumping part of the heart cycle (systole) and can be due to the opening of abnormally stiff aortic and pulmonic valves (which is usually not heard) or due to the closing sound of an abnormal mitral valve.

Snaps: Snaps can be heard in the resting part of the heart cycle (diastole) and are usually due to the opening of an abnormal mitral valve.

Bruit (BROO-EE): Besides listening directly to the heart, a doctor will sometimes listen to the arteries in the neck or the arteries in the abdomen which supply blood to the kidneys. In normal arteries one would hear nothing. However, if some part of the artery is partially blocked, you can sometimes hear the blood moving past a blockage. This sound is called a bruit.

3. Feeling (Palpation):

Pulses: In assessing the left side of the heart, one can feel the pulses, as described earlier and determine something about the rate and rhythm of the heart beat. **[See Figure 3A]** Feeling carefully along the neck to the side of the windpipe (trachea), the carotid pulses are easily detected. Be careful to feel only lightly so as not to irritate or block the vessel, and only feel on one side at a time so as not to block blood flow to the brain. See if you can find your own carotid pulsations. The normal pulse has a brisk upstroke, followed by a rapid downstroke and a pause.

Liver: In addition to feeling the carotid pulses, the doctor palpates the abdomen to see if the liver is enlarged. When the right side of the heart fails, blood gets backed up and the liver becomes engorged and swollen.

Heart: The heart should also be felt directly to see what can be learned from feeling it as it beats. When the doctor places the palm of his hand on the left side of your chest, she or he is feeling for two things. The first is the point where the heart can be felt to beat with the greatest intensity. This point is called the point of maximum intensity (PMI) and is usually located near the left nipple. (See if you can feel yours while laying down, if not, try lying to the left side). The PMI is normally the size of a quarter. The second thing the doctor feels for is a movement next to the breastbone. Normally, this is not felt, but if the right side of the heart is abnormally large, it can be felt to push up or "heave" against the breastbone (sternum) during the heartbeat.

The doctor can use the tips of her or his fingers to feel the pulses in the neck, elbow, wrist, groin, behind the knee and the feet. This assures that blood is reaching all of the extremities. A doctor may also attempt to feel the largest artery, the aorta, as it passes down through the abdominal area. In relatively thin people, this can usually be felt. Sometimes, the examiner can also estimate the size of this artery. When it is thought to be larger than 4 cms., further investigation is needed to assure that the artery is not abnormally ballooned out or dilated. Such an abnormally dilated aorta is called an aneurysm and, if large enough, it is in danger of bursting or rupturing.

4. Tapping (Percussion): Tapping is rarely used to assess the size of the heart. By tapping with the middle finger of the right hand on the middle finger of the left hand as it rests on the chest wall, a physician can hear different sounds, depending on what is below the chest wall at that point. By tapping from the left side of the chest toward the middle, the doctor can get a crude estimate of the heart's size. Today, however, most doctors use a chest x-ray for this purpose since it is much more accurate.

C. Additional tests: An electrocardiogram (EKG) and a chest x-ray are sometimes used to complete the heart examination. Again, this is usually only necessary when symptoms or findings on the physical examination warrant further investigation.

Chest x-ray: This is a picture of the soft tissues and bony structures of the chest, and enables measurement of the size of the heart. Occasionally, an enlarged chamber can also be seen on the x-ray.

EKG: Essentially, an EKG is an electrical picture of the heart. It shows what electrical impulses are generated and transmitted during the pumping cycle of the heart. It is excellent for determining the various complicated rhythms of the heart, but it is also useful in determining if any chambers of the heart are enlarged, or if any of the heart muscle is dying from lack of oxygen because the small vessels which supply blood to the heart itself are blocked (as happens in a heart attack).

The Echocardiogram: The echocardiogram is just an ultrasound picture of the heart (visualization through sound waves). Echocardiograms are good for seeing exactly what is wrong with a diseased heart valve, for seeing how big the chambers are, how thick the heart muscle is, and for determining the pumping efficiency of the heart.

Arteriogram: An arteriogram is an x-ray dye study of the heart. The arteriogram gives an exact map of the arteries around the heart. These arteries supply blood to the muscle of the heart and blockages in these arteries are the main cause of heart attacks. With the help of the arteriogram, the doctor can tell exactly where blockages are and plan various treatments, which may include surgery. The doctor can also determine how the valves are working with this study. Regurgitation of blood through valves and holes in the heart wall may cause the heart to fail because it is having to pump too large a volume of fluid. Any amount of blood that escapes backward through a valve must be pumped through again (twice), and this is very inefficient and overworks the heart from a volume standpoint. Blood passing through a narrowed valve, on the other hand, overworks the heart in a different way. To pump blood through a narrowed valve, the heart must generate greater pressures, which causes the heart to be overworked from a pressure standpoint.

CHAPTER 7

The Chest and Lungs

The function of the lungs is to exchange gases between the blood and the atmosphere. As our bodies break down the food we eat into energy that can be used by the cells, oxygen is used and carbon dioxide is created by the tissues. These two gases must be exchanged every minute in order for us to stay alive. The brain controls the rate and depth of our breathing in such a way as to maintain adequate gaseous exchange. The brain's drive to breathe is controlled by the level of carbon dioxide in the blood. As this level increases (such as during exercise), we breathe faster in order to exchange more carbon dioxide from our lungs into the atmosphere. If we did not breathe faster, the carbon dioxide dissolved in our blood would cause the blood to become more acidic and our bodies do not function well with more than the normal amount of acid.

As we exercise we also require more oxygen. However, the increased rate or depth of breathing needed to eliminate the excess carbon dioxide is usually more than enough to supply the extra oxygen needed. Only in certain abnormal circumstances is the rate and depth of breathing controlled by the level of oxygen in the blood.

If we were unable to eliminate enough carbon dioxide from our lungs over a period of several hours or days, our kidneys would begin to compensate. They would sense that the acid in the blood was building up and would hold on to more base (or alkaline) than usual in order to keep the level of acid in the blood at the normal level. So the lungs control the exchange of oxygen and the lungs and kidneys together control the exchange of carbon dioxide, and hence acid.

The mechanism of gas exchange: The lungs are enclosed in the chest wall. In order for air to enter them, the pressure inside the lungs must be less than the atmospheric pressure outside the lungs, since gas flows from high pressure to low pressure just as water flows downhill. When we breathe, our chest wall expands and our diaphragm moves down, creating a negative pressure in the lungs which then sucks air into them. When we exhale, our chest wall relaxes and the air flows out as the pressure in the lungs exceeds the atmospheric pressure outside.

The purpose of examining the chest and lungs is for the doctor to see if adequate gas exchange is occurring. As with the examination of the other organ systems, the doctor has four methods at her or his disposal: to look, listen, feel and tap.

1. Looking (Inspection): When examining the patient, the physician's first question should be: is this person exchanging enough oxygen and carbon dioxide? The second question should be: is this person having to work very hard to exchange the proper amount of gases?

A person who is sitting comfortably in the office is most likely exchanging enough of these gases. On the other hand, the person who is short of breath, breathing very fast and sweating profusely is probably not exchanging enough gases.

The amount of gas exchanged by the lungs is equal to the rate of breathing times the amount (or volume) of each breath. To assess how much gas exchange is occurring the doctor must look at both the rate and the depth of breathing. Adults breathe anywhere between 12 and 20 times per minute, and children breathe much faster. When problems occur and the body needs to exchange more gases, the breathing rate may go up, the depth of breathing may increase, or both. At other times, problems such as injury may cause breathing to be painful. In these circumstances, a person may begin to take more shallow breaths (in order to have less pain), and have to breathe faster in order to compensate and exchange an adequate amount of gases.

The work of breathing must also be tested. For example, when a person is unable to exchange adequate gases or becomes exhausted when trying to do so, respiratory failure is occurring and this constitutes an emergency. Treatment could be as simple as oxygen therapy or as complicated as placing them on a machine to breathe for them until they have improved.

By looking at the patient, the doctor can get information which is valuable in deciding what the problem is and how to treat it. When a person has great difficulty breathing, they begin to use additional muscles to help them expand their chest wall. Muscles in the neck, which are not usually used to breathe, are asked by the brain to join in the fight to get more air. As the body exerts great force to generate large negative pressure in the lungs (to suck more air in), some parts of the chest wall collapse as they are sucked in by this large pressure. For example, a person with great difficulty breathing may have retractions (or indented areas) in between the ribs, or above the collar bone. Their stomach may move inward with breathing instead of outward as usual. In babies, the nostrils may flare out while breathing -- all these are signs to the observant doctor that difficulty in breathing is occurring and that treatment is needed.

In addition, the doctor should always observe the movement of the chest wall to see if the movement is symmetrical (the same on both sides). As the lungs expand, both sides of the chest wall should move together. If not, this could be a clue to what the problem is.

The doctor should also look for any deformities of the chest wall which may have been present since birth or may be due to injury or growth of tumors.

2. Listening (Auscultation): In the examination of the chest, the stethoscope is particularly important, because the sounds that can be heard are often a clue to what is going on inside.

Several sounds may be heard when listening to the chest, some of which are mentioned on the next page.

Bronchial and vesicular breath sounds are the names given to two types of normal lung sounds. In both, the sound heard is due to air moving freely through the airways in the lungs. The pitch and quality of these sounds are different, but they are both normal and heard in most patients.

An additional method of assessing breath sounds is to note whether they are normal or decreased in volume or amount. A decrease in the amount of normal breath sounds could mean that very little air is actually entering or leaving the lungs and that the person is in respiratory failure, even if other abnormal breath sounds are not present.

Some types of abnormal breath sounds:

Rales are sounds best described as crackles, since they sound somewhat like the crackling of Rice Crispies in a bowl. Rales are heard when small portions of the airways which have collapsed during expiration are suddenly opened by the force of incoming air. Rales are almost always abnormal and can be due to such problems as pneumonia or fluid overload.

Rhonchi are coarse sounds heard on expiration. They are due to the presence of fluid in some of the airways. As the air is forced out past the fluid, the fluid gurgles and rhonchi are heard.

Wheezes are high pitched whistling sounds usually heard on expiration. They indicate that the airways are narrowed, and as air is forced through them, a whistling sound is created. Wheezing can be heard in asthma, chronic obstructive pulmonary disease and in some allergic reactions, and is an indication that additional work of breathing is being expended to rid the lungs of air.

Rubs are heard when the two covering surfaces of the lung are inflamed and rub against one another. Usually these surfaces are smooth and have a lubricating fluid in-between them. However, in some infections which affect the lining of the lungs, this smoothness disappears and a rub is heard.

Stridor is a high pitched sound that comes from the throat when air is being drawn into the lungs while the vocal chords are not fully open. This sound may be heard when the tissues of the throat are abnormally swollen. This sound may indicate respiratory failure.

Egophony is a term describing the change in sound that may occur when lung tissue is no longer filled with air, but becomes fluid filled. A patient may be asked to say "ee" while the doctor listens. If the area of the lung being examined is fluid-filled because of disease, then the "ee" sound will change to sound like"aa".

3. Feeling (Palpation): Looking and feeling go hand in hand, and many of the same abnormalities which were seen can also be felt. Doctors typically feel the movement of the chest wall during breathing to make sure that both sides are moving equally well. If one side moves less than the other it could mean that the diaphragm (muscle of breathing) is paralyzed. A doctor typically places her or his hands on a patient's back at symmetrical positions on either side, and feels as the patient breathes. In addition, a doctor may press on a certain area of the chest wall to see if it is tender or if there is any evidence of injury or broken ribs. A broken rib is often tender at the site of the break. This is however difficult to distinguish from other causes of tenderness over a small area. In order to confirm that a broken rib is causing the problem, the doctor may press on the front and back of the chest wall simultaneously. Since ribs are bow-shaped, pressing from both ends (front and back of the body) will cause the broken area (if there is one) to be painful just as if it were being directly compressed. If the rib is not broken, this will not be painful at all.

The sound of the voice is transmitted through the resonant air-filled lung tissue and can be felt as a vibration on the skin. Try this: place the palm of your hand on someone's bare back and ask them to say: "ninety-nine". You should feel the vibration of their voice in your hand. This is called vocal fremitus and can be either increased or decreased in certain diseases. In pneumonia, when part of the lung is filled with blood and pus instead of air, the sound is transmitted more efficiently to the skin and fremitus is increased. When fluid has filled the space between the lung and the chest wall, the sound is transmitted less efficiently and the fremitus is decreased. This occurs in such conditions as heart failure and some types of lung cancer.

4. Percussion (tapping): In examining the lungs, the doctor may tap over the chest wall in much the same way as she or he does when examining the abdomen. The sound which is heard helps to determine the state of the tissues below and can be very useful in diagnosis.

If the sound over one side is like a high pitched drum (tympanitic), while the sound over the other lung is normal or hollow sounding, it might mean that one lung has collapsed inside the chest wall and has a leak. If so, this is potentially a serious and even life-threatening condition that demands immediate treatment.

In the same way that fluid collections in the chest cavity (around the lungs) can be detected by feeling the absence or presence of fremitus, fluid can sometimes be detected by tapping over both sides of the chest wall. On the normal side, the sound will be hollow or resonant signifying that air-filled tissue is beneath the tapping finger. On the side with a fluid collection, the sound will be more dull at the bottom of the lung where the fluid has collected around it. You can confirm that it is fluid by having the patient lay down on her or his side. The level of fluid will move to the side which is down, and the dull sound will no longer be at the bottom of the chest wall at the back, but will now be at the side of the chest wall.

Fluid collections are not the only things that cause the tapped sound to be dull. Lung tissue that has collapsed and is no longer air-filled can also cause a dull sound, as can lung tissue that is infected and has become filled with blood and pus -- as commonly occurs in pneumonia.

Additional lung tests, the chest x-ray: is a typical part of the medical examination for any patients with lung or heart problems. It allows the doctor to see a black and white image of the lung tissue, the heart, and the bones of the chest wall and spinal column. It is extremely useful for the evaluation of conditions such as pneumonia, heart failure, asthma, emphysema and lung cancer. It is widely used because it is relatively inexpensive and yields such a large amount of information.

The arterial blood gas is a blood test that is obtained from an artery. It tells the doctor about the composition of the blood as it comes out of the heart. It is useful in determining the oxygen content of the blood, the carbon dioxide content of the blood and the pH (or acid) content of the blood. It tells us how well the lungs are doing at exchanging gases, and if the kidneys have come into play to help the lungs. In addition, it tells the doctor what percentage of the oxygen carrying molecules in the blood are fully saturated with oxygen.

Pulse oximetry is another quick and easy way of determining the percentage of the oxygen carrying molecules in the blood and if they are fully saturated with oxygen.

Pulmonary function tests are performed in a laboratory and give very specific details about the function of the lungs both normally and in the diseased state. A patient is connected to a complicated breathing machine and asked to do certain respiratory maneuvers such as breathe in and out as fast and deeply as possible. A computer then analyzes the gases that go in and out of the patient's lungs, and it is able to quantify the performance of the patient in relation to normal, healthy persons.

CHAPTER 8

The Abdomen

Examination of the abdomen is quick and painless, and yields a great deal of information. **[Figure 8A]** Since only obvious deformities in the size or shape of the abdomen can be detected by observation, the physician's methods of palpation, auscultation and percussion become relatively more important for the abdominal examination. Examination of the digestive (or gastrointestinal) system also includes an examination of the kidneys as well as the urinary and circulatory systems. In women, this procedure includes an examination of the reproductive system.

A. Correct Positioning: A patient's abdomen is best examined with the patient lying on his or her back, with hands to the side and legs slightly bent at the knees. This position is best for relaxing the muscles of the abdominal wall and allowing the doctor to palpate the deep organs more easily.

The organs of the abdomen are located in the same position in nearly every patient. The symptoms for certain diseases have classic locations where people often describe their discomfort or pain as originating. For this reason, doctors have to think about which organs or diseases cause pain in particular regions. **[Figure 8B]**

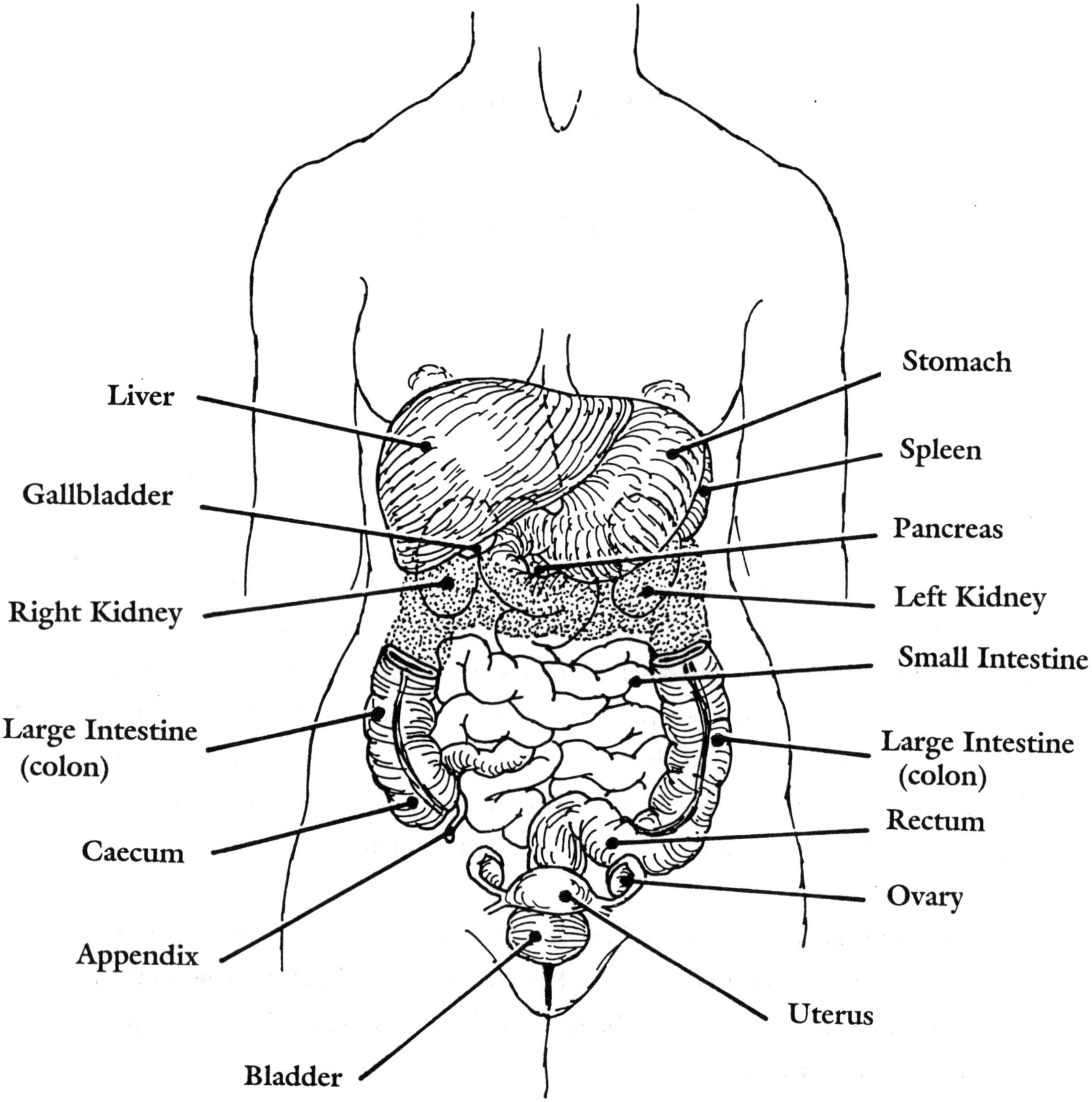

EVALUATION OF THE ABDOMEN

Figure 8A

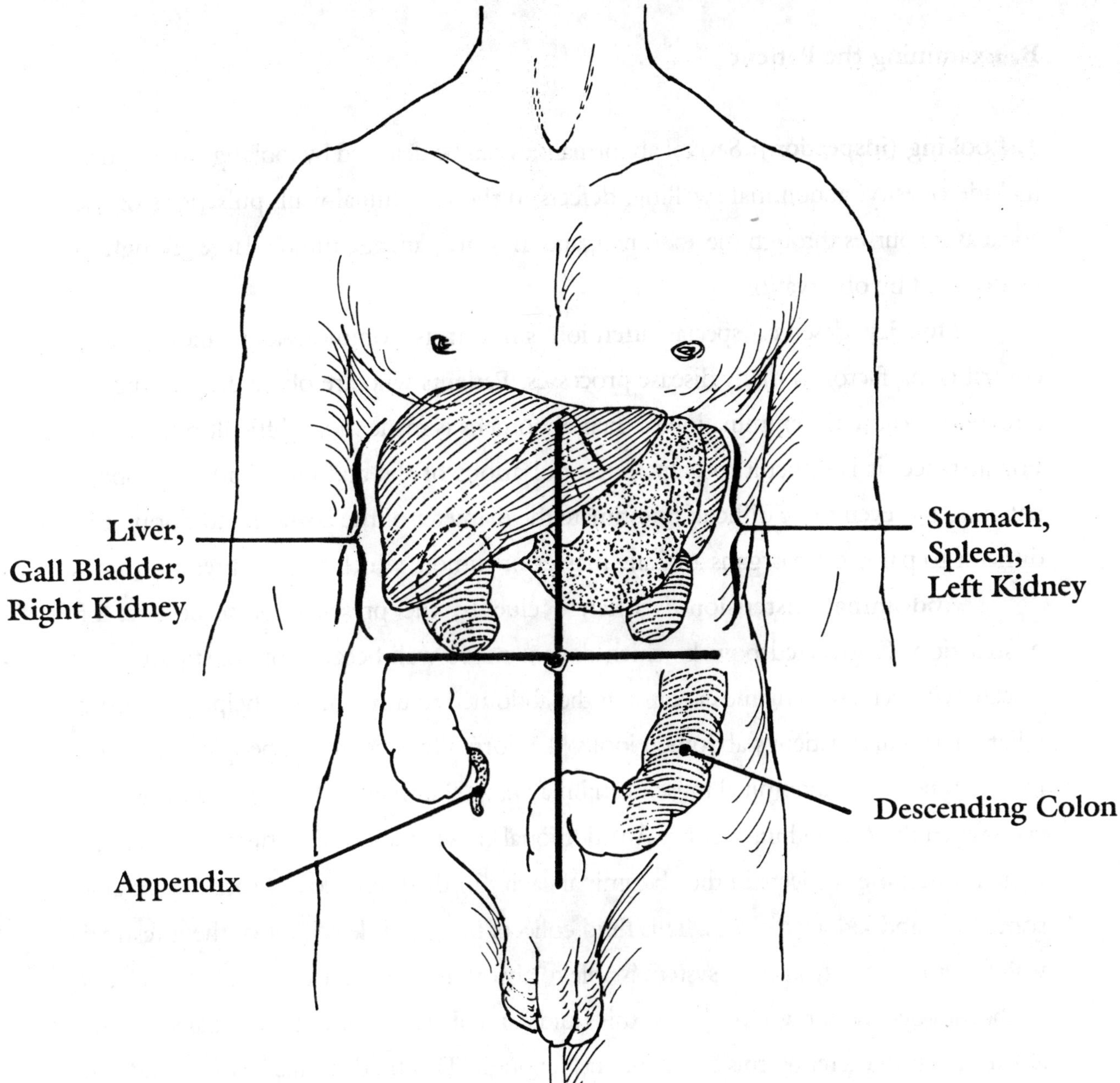

QUADRANTS OF THE ABDOMEN

Figure 8B

B. Examining the Patient

1. Looking (inspection): Several abnormalities can be detected by looking alone. These include obesity, abdominal swelling, defects in the abdominal wall, pulsations of the aorta as it courses through the abdomen, and in some patients, tumors large enough to be detected by observation.

Obesity deserves special attention since it is common and since it is a contributing factor to many disease processes. Patients who are obese deserve special attention because the examination of their abdomens is made more difficult by obesity. For instance, it is difficult to palpate the pulsations of the abdominal aorta in obese patients, and even more difficult to estimate the diameter of the aorta. In addition, it is difficult to palpate the organs and any masses or tumors which may be present.

Abdominal distension is often a clue to the presence of some sort of obstruction. Obstructed bowels which do not move well because of constipation or disease will increase in diameter, causing the abdomen to distend. It is helpful to know what a particular patient's abdomen looks like normally, since some people have poor muscle tone in the abdominal muscles and may have abdomens which appear distended even when there is nothing wrong. An additional cause of abdominal distension is fluid which sometimes collects in the abdominal cavity in the presence of heart disease and some liver and kidney diseases. This fluid collects because it leaks out of the intestinal wall faster than the lymphatic system is able to absorb it. In addition, if the heart is weak or the kidneys are not working well, this fluid can collect because these organs are not able to assist in excreting this extra fluid fast enough. This fluid is called ascites, and can collect in large enough quantities to cause abdominal distension.

Defects in the muscles of the abdominal wall, called hernias, can occasionally be seen by inspection alone, but are usually detected and best evaluated by palpation. These defects can be congenital (present at birth) or acquired after birth (as a result of abdominal surgery) and are usually not painful. There are several types, some of which will be discussed in a later chapter. Hernias, in general, pose no immediate threat, but since at times the intestines can bulge into the hernia and get blocked off, most doctors prefer to repair hernias on an elective basis. The exception to this is the umbilical or "belly button" hernia, which is fairly common in children. Some umbilical hernias resolve on their own, so many doctors prefer to wait and see if this happens first. If it does not disappear, surgery can always be done at a later date.

Finally, there are some observations which can be made only rarely, but these are very important and should never be missed. In patients with severe pancreatitis (inflamation of the pancreas), for example, blood which leaks out of the pancreas is visible through the abdominal wall. This accumulated blood appears as a bluish/gray discoloration of the skin surrounding the flanks or umbilicus (belly button). This indicates that the pancreatitis is severe enough to have caused tissue death and bleeding. Another such important observation can be made in some patients with advanced liver failure due to cirrhosis. In this condition, blood has difficulty passing through the normal vessels in the liver, so it gets backed up and tries to reach the heart by alternate routes. One such route is for the blood to flow into the veins which are in the skin surrounding the umbilicus, and to cause them to become dilated (enlarged) and visible on the skin as bluish-gray, snake-like discolorations. Since they are seen radiating like snakes from the center of the umbilicus, doctors have nicknamed this finding "caput Medusae" after the Greek god Medusa who had snakes in her hair.

2. Listening (Auscultation): For most parts of the physical examination, doctors feel that auscultation should be conducted last. However, in the case of the abdominal examination, most doctors feel that auscultation should be done first, before the normal resting state of the abdominal organs have been changed by palpation. For example, the bowel sounds of a person might be more or less active after deep palpation than before.

Listening to the abdomen with a stethoscope reveals the presence or absence of bowel sounds, which are the continuous and regular movements of the stomach and the small and large intestines. All of us have heard a stomach "growl" or "rumble" and these are merely the normal sounds that food makes as it passes through the gastrointestinal system. Normal bowel sounds are the gurglings which can be heard several times per minute, as waves of peristalsis (muscular contractions) pass down through the walls of the intestines. Abnormal bowel sounds are simply too many, or too few, of the normal bowel sounds. Hyperactive bowel sounds occur when patients have diarrhea, for example, or when the intestines are in the early phase of obstruction. In the beginning of intestinal obstruction, the bowels move frequently and vigorously to try and get the contents of the intestines around the obstructed area. This sounds like hyperactive bowel sounds which are often of a higher pitch than normal bowel sounds.

When no bowel sounds are heard after listening for one minute, the patient is said to have ileus, which means that the normal waves of peristalsis have ceased altogether. Common causes of ileus include peritonitis (inflamation in the abdominal cavity) and post-operative recovery from abdominal surgery (after the bowels have been manipulated during surgery, it takes several days for them to recover and start to function normally again).

In addition to listening to bowel sounds, the abdomen should be auscultated for the presence of bruits, which are the rushing sounds made by abnormal blood flow. Abdominal bruits are occasionally heard in the aorta and the renal arteries and suggest narrowing of the vessels due to atherosclerosis. It is important to examine for these since they may be a sign of early atherosclerosis. Also, if the renal artery is stenosed (narrowed) it could be causing a form of high blood pressure which is often curable!

3. Feeling (Palpation): Palpation of the abdomen yields a lot of useful information. There are several ways to palpate the abdomen: with one hand, with one hand on top of the other, and with one hand in front and one on the back of the patient.

The one-handed method is the most widely used, and is good for examining the internal organs such as the stomach, liver, spleen and intestines. The two-handed method is used to augment the one handed method, and is especially good for examining the deep organs such as the kidneys. In the two-handed method, the doctor palpates directly with his or her dominant or preferred hand while pressing over this hand with the other hand. It is thought by some that by applying pressure with the other hand, the dominant hand is better able to feel abnormalities. The method with one hand in front and the other at the back is also useful to palpate deep organs, which can occasionally be felt between the two hands as they press in towards one another.

Generally, doctors palpate in all four quadrants to see if any organs can be identified. Usually, no organs are felt at all, and this can be entirely normal! In fact, it is more disturbing to feel organs than to feel nothing at all. Most often the liver can be felt if the doctor presses down during the patient's inspiration. This is entirely normal, but if the liver is felt, its size should be estimated to ensure that it is not enlarged. With special movements and deep palpation the spleen and kidneys can occasionally be palpated, but if the spleen, kidneys or bladder are palpated on routine abdominal examination, this is considered to be abnormal. A palpable spleen in an adult means it is abnormally large, as are palpable kidneys. If the bladder is palpated, this means that it is quite full, or possibly that an obstruction is preventing it from emptying. Similarly, if the uterus of a woman can be palpated, then it is abnormally large.

Feeling the liver: The liver can usually be palpated during deep inspiration, and it feels like a soft but firm mass located in the right upper quadrant. It can sometimes be abnormally small or firm in diseases such as cirrhosis. At other times it can be tender to palpation such as in hepatitis or right-sided heart failure. Sometimes masses can be felt in the liver and numerous types of tumors become considerations in the diagnosis. If the liver can be palpated then its size should be measured, using percussion to determine if it is enlarged. Enlarged livers are seen in many diseases. Occasionally the gallbladder can be felt in patients with gallstones or cholecystitis (an inflamed, enlarged gallbladder). The gallbladder is located below the lower edge of the liver.

Feeling the spleen: The spleen is not normally felt at all. If assessing the size of the spleen is important in a particular patient, she or he can be asked to roll slightly toward the right side, which will cause the spleen (located in the left upper quadrant) to fall forward and downward, making it easier and more likely to be felt. Enlarged spleens can be seen in many diseases such as infections, connective tissue disorders, lymphomas, leukemia, portal hypertension or cirrhosis.

Feeling the kidneys: Again, the kidneys can not usually be palpated except in very thin persons and in infants. The kidneys should be palpated for normal size in the examination of all infants because of two childhood diseases: polycystic kidney disease (kidneys with balloon type cysts) and Wilm's tumor which is a relatively common form of childhood cancer.

Palpating for masses: A physician should always feel for masses (tumors) in all quadrants. Masses can occasionally be palpated in the liver, pancreas, stomach, small intestines, large intestine, bladder, uterus, ovaries and kidneys.

Palpating for pulsations: In thin individuals, the aorta can be seen to pulsate as it passes through the abdomen. In most individuals its pulsations can be palpated, and an estimate of its size should be made. If an abdominal aorta is felt to be greater than 4-5 cms in diameter, then further diagnostic workup is indicated to rule out an abdominal aortic aneurysm -- which is a dangerous ballooning or dilation of the aorta -- which can be treated and even surgically repaired if necessary.

In addition to the pulsations of the aorta, the liver can, on rare occasions, be felt to pulsate. This usually indicates that there is an abnormality with the right side of the heart, usually the tricuspid valve.

4. Tapping (Percussion): Percussion of the abdomen is done primarily to determine the size of the liver and spleen, and to determine if an abnormal collection of fluid exists in the abdominal cavity.

The size of the liver is estimated in the following way. The doctor percusses, beginning over the right lung near the nipple, where a flat or slightly tympanitic sound is heard. As the percussing hand moves downward over the liver, the sound changes to being dull. Below the level of the liver the sound again becomes tympanitic, indicating that the hollow organs such as the large and small intestines are being percussed. The area of dullness corresponds to the size of the liver, and liver enlargement can be a clue to many disease processes.

The spleen can be percussed in a similar way, except that the patient needs to be in the left lateral decubitus position -- which is laying on the back, rolled slightly to the left side, but not all the way onto the side. In this position, the spleen is located against the abdominal wall and can be percussed more easily. Beginning over the left lung the percussing hands move down over the dull area which represents the spleen. At the lower edge of the spleen, tympanitic sounds return, indicating that hollow organs (such as bowel) are beneath. In this way, the size of the spleen is measured.

Finally, percussion is used to determine the presence of ascites -- an abnormal collection of fluid in the abdominal cavity, but outside of the organs themselves. If fluid has collected in the peritoneal cavity, it will locate at the bottom of that cavity due to gravity. The air-filled bowels will float on top of it. If one were to percuss someone with ascites beginning at the flank (lower back) and moving upwards toward the umbilicus (navel), one would notice a transition zone where the flat sound of percussing over the fluid was replaced by the tympanitic sound of percussing over the bowels. This would be the level of fluid in the peritoneum. In order to prove that the dullness was not a solid organ, but was indeed due to fluid levels, the doctor could then turn the patient onto her or his side and percuss again. Since the bowels would float up to the uppermost side of the abdominal wall and the fluid would sink to the lower flank, the area of dullness would shift just as the fluid had shifted. This would confirm to the doctor the presence of ascites.

One additional application of percussion in the abdominal examination involves percussing the back to see if the kidneys may be irritated and painful. Doctors usually tap with a fist over the lower back just to the side of the spine and just below the last rib. This is not normally painful but may be extremely painful if the kidneys are infected. The patient may not have noticed this pain since it is related to sudden motion (the tapping of the fist), especially if the patient has been inactive.

F. The Rectal Examination: An important part of the abdominal examination is the rectal examination. It is usually conducted with the patient in the fetal (curled up) position, but can also be comfortably conducted with the patient standing and bending over a table (in women, the rectal examination is often included as the final part of a pelvic examination in the standard position for a pelvic exam).

Information gained through the rectal examination, in both men and women, includes assessing the tone of the sphincter (muscle which closes off the anus) -- which is especially important in patients with neurological complaints or problems with holding in their stool. Also, the end of the rectum can be palpated for polyps, which are abnormal growths that can become cancerous. A small sample of stool which inevitably remains on the doctor's glove can be tested instantly for the presence of undetected blood.

In men, the rectal examination is useful for assessing the size of the prostate gland and whether any abnormal growths are located in the prostate. Prostate disease is one of the most common problems in aging men. Two conditions predominate: 1)In benign hypertrophy of the prostate the normal tissue of the aging prostate overgrows and the prostate becomes enlarged. Since the tube that conveys urine from the bladder through the shaft of the penis must pass through the prostate, an enlarged prostate can block this tube and make it difficult for men to urinate or to empty their bladders completely. This is why most older men have a weaker stream of urine or may dribble more than younger men, and why many men have to get up several times at night and empty their bladders. Certain medication can often be taken to shrink the prostate gland. Surgery is sometimes required to remove the blockage. 2)In cancer of the prostate, nodules or growths are felt in the outer border of the prostate. When present, these need to be sampled to see if cancer cells are present. Most prostate cancer occurs in very old men and it rarely spreads fast. For men who are diagnosed with cancer of the prostate, most will die of some other cause before the prostate cancer kills them. If found early, or in a younger man, the cancer usually responds well to surgical removal and chemotherapy.

In women, the rectal examination is useful to assess for a rectocele, a condition where part of the rectum bulges into the vagina.

G. Peritonitis: The organs inside the abdominal cavity are each surrounded by a thin membrane called the visceral peritoneum. Similarly, the abdominal wall itself is surrounded by a thin membrane called the parietal peritoneum. These membranes are normally very close together and separated by a small amount of fluid, which is normally present for lubrication as the intestines move. (Imagine a long garden hose stuffed inside a garbage bag which is filled with water. The inner lining of the garbage bag would be the parietal peritoneum and the outer wall of the hose would be the visceral peritoneum. The water in the bag, which the hose is lying in, represents the fluid that is present in small quantities in our abdominal cavities.)

Sometimes an abnormal amount of fluid collects in the potential space in the abdomen -- just as if extra fluid collected in the garbage bag. This is called ascites and is an abnormal amount, or type, of fluid which collects in the potential space between the visceral and parietal membranes. Irritation of these membranes leads to inflammation and is very painful. Whenever one of the hollow organs perforates (such as a ruptured appendix or a perforated ulcer -- just like the hose breaking inside the bag), the contents of the bowels (food) spill into the peritoneal space and cause severe pain. Such patients are said to have peritonitis (inflammation of the peritoneum) and are almost always in need of emergency surgery. When peritonitis occurs, the bowels stop moving completely and any movement or stretching of the peritoneal membranes causes extreme pain. For this reason, the abdominal muscles contract involuntarily and the abdomen becomes rigid. There are several classic and easy signs of peritonitis which doctors routinely check for in very ill patients.

1. Absent bowel sounds: the bowels have stopped moving altogether.
2. Guarding: the patient has so much pain from the irritation of the peritoneal membranes that their abdominal muscles are contracted, and it is difficult to feel any other abdominal structures on examination.

3. Rebound tenderness: any movement or stretching of the membranes causes severe pain. For instance, if the doctor presses firmly but gently and then rapidly withdraws his or her hand, this causes the membrane to suddenly stretch back into its original position -- and produces pain in the patient's abdomen. Similarly, even jiggling the bed would cause pain for the same reason.

If any patient has evidence of these signs, she or he is said to have peritoneal signs and needs evaluation by a surgeon.

H. Location of pain: As a doctor examines the abdomen of a patient, the location of their pain is very useful in determining possible causes. This is too detailed and complex a problem to discuss fully here, but common types will be discussed briefly as examples.

Pancreatic pain: Usually located above the umbilicus (belly button) in the middle of the abdomen and often radiates to the back.

Spleen pain: Usually located in the left upper quadrant and may radiate to the left shoulder.

Pain of diverticulitis: Pain from diverticulitis (abnormal outpouchings of the large intestinal wall which periodically become inflamed) and is often located in the right or left lower quadrant of the abdomen.

Kidney pain: Often located in the flanks (lower back) and may radiate into the groin.

Pain from appendicitis: This pain is usually located around the umbilicus at first and then moves into the lower right quadrant as the condition worsens.

Intestinal pain: Usually crampy in nature and can be located almost anywhere.

When abnormalities are detected, additional tests may often be needed to make an accurate diagnosis. The imaging studies which are commonly used to evaluate the abdomen are ultrasound (sound waves), CAT (computed axial tomography, or computerized x-ray from many locations in the area), scanning (picture taken of radioactive substances injected into the patient which accumulates in the organ) and MRI (magnetic resonance imaging: means of creating images using magnetism).

CHAPTER 9

The Arms, Legs and Joints

A complete physical examination includes an inspection of the arms, legs, and their joints. In addition, the neck and back should be carefully examined, especially when a person's complaint may be related to muscular or skeletal problems. For this part of the physical examination the physician relies primarily on the procedures of looking and feeling, since listening and tapping are not of as much value.

A. Looking: In general, the arms and legs should appear symmetrical. Usually one foot or hand is minimally larger than the other and this is normal, especially if that side is the dominant or most often used side. Similarly, the muscles should be roughly the same size on both sides of the body. If there is any doubt, the circumference of both sides should be measured. The muscles of both upper and lower extremities should be carefully observed for signs of wasting, which could be signs of general weight loss from any number of conditions, or could be signs of specific muscle or nervous system diseases. The muscles should be observed for small twitch-like movements (called fasiculations), which can be signs that the nerves which supply them are no longer functioning properly. The patient should be asked about any problems with coordination of their movements and they should be observed doing simple movements with their hands and arms to see whether the movement is fluid and well-coordinated. An observation of a patient walking, for example, can often reveal much information about the type of disease which may be causing the problem, and may give evidence as to whether the problem is in the muscles, joints, nerves or brain.

B. Feeling: Next, it is important for the physician to feel the muscles and joints of the arms and legs because valuable discoveries can be made which were not evident to the eye. Careful survey of all the muscle beds should be made with careful note to any swellings or tender areas. Swollen areas could be bruised or infected tissue, lymph nodes or even tumors. Tender areas could be caused by some of the same things mentioned above or could be due to injury. In addition, tender areas should be further examined to determine if the tenderness corresponds to bone, muscle, tendons or ligaments. Tendons connect muscles to bones while ligaments connect bones to bones. This may help the doctor to tell what caused the problem and be better able to treat it.

Examining the Joints: [Figure 9A] Joints are examined by looking and feeling. When a doctor is called upon to examine a joint, it is usually because of a complaint of pain on the part of the patient. Joints can be painful because of a large variety of problems, including injury, various types of arthritis, local infections, generalized body diseases, and even spread of infections from other parts of the body. It is important to distinguish the cause of a painful joint because early treatment can relieve symptoms and often save the patient from long-lasting complications.

A joint which is painful should be evaluated immediately. First, the doctor should find out if any injury occurred and at what times of day or with what types of activity the joint is most painful. The joint should be observed and palpated while it is in motion. Observation of a moving joint will often reveal at what point in the joint's movement the most pain occurs. Feeling the joint will further identify if the motion is smooth and whether or not the joint is grating or gets stuck at certain positions. Joints, too, can be painful because of bone, tendon or ligament problems, and the cause should always be sought.

If a joint is swollen, it is sometimes because the tissues surrounding it are injured and swollen, but it is usually because extra fluid is present in the joint. The fluid may be blood, pus, or an abnormal amount of joint fluid which has accumulated due to inflammation. Usually palpation will reveal whether a joint is swollen because the surrounding tissues are swollen, or because the joint has fluid in it. When a joint does

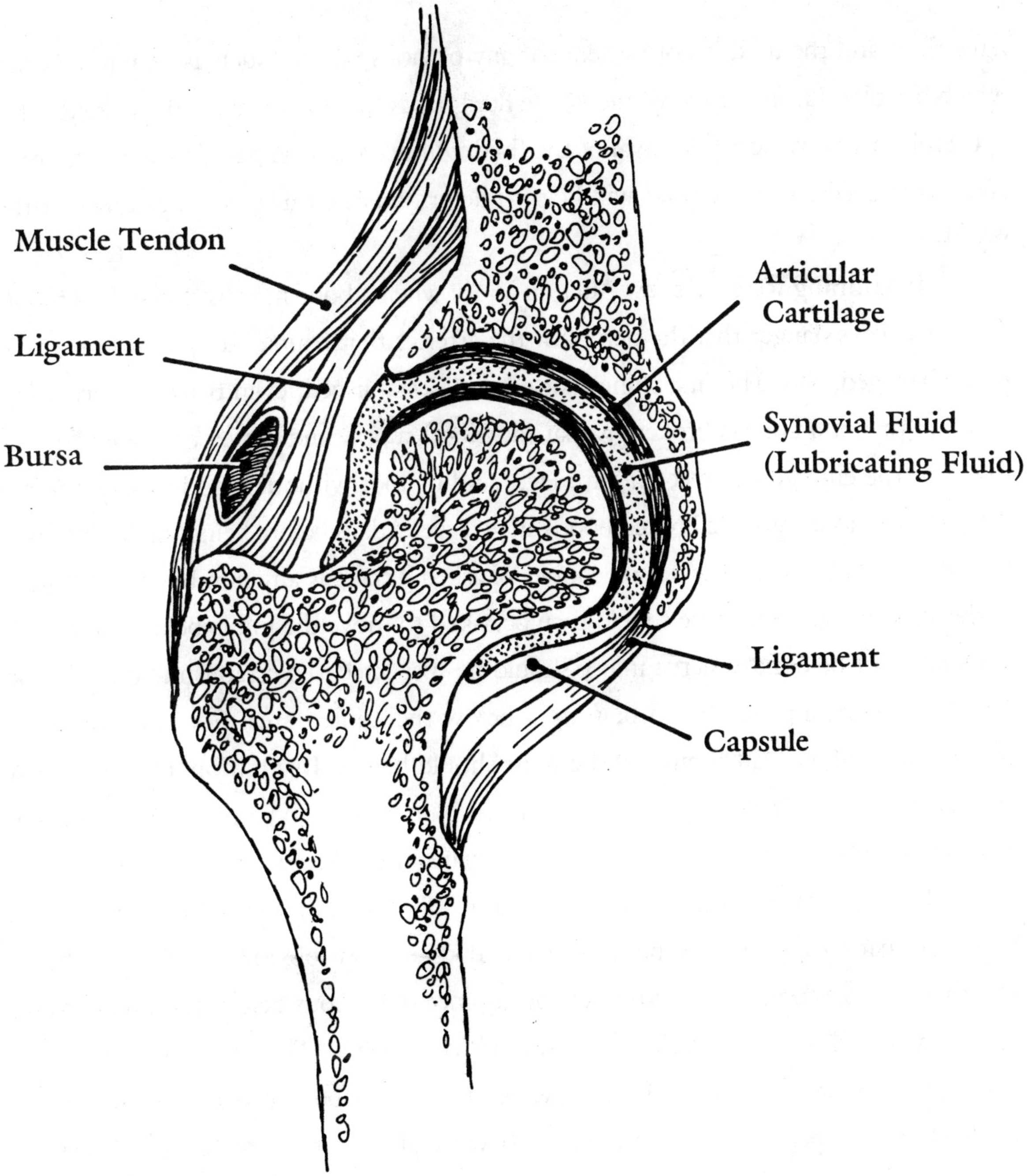

THE JOINT

Figure 9A

have fluid and the fluid is not present for any obvious reason (such as an injured knee which has blood from a torn ligament) the fluid needs to be removed and analyzed. This is useful for two reasons: removal of the fluid will decrease the pain in the joint, and a laboratory analysis of the fluid will help to determine the cause and treatment of the problem.

Examining for fractures: After an injury when a bone may have been fractured, there is always danger that the nerves or the arteries that course along that bone have been damaged, too. The first thing that must be established, even before determining whether or not a bone is broken, is that the blood supply and nerves are intact. If not, this is a true emergency since an arm, leg, hand or foot without blood supply will die within a few hours, while a broken bone can go several days before being set. To establish that the nerves are intact the person should be asked if there is any numbness or tingling in the affected part. She or he should then be asked to move the joints below the injury. If this cannot be done, a nerve injury should be suspected. To establish that the blood supply is intact, a pulse should be sought below the injured area. For instance, if the elbow is injured, the radial pulse in the wrist should be felt. In addition, the area below the injury should stay warm and pink. If it turns blue or cold and a pulse cannot be felt, an arterial injury should be suspected -- immediate surgical repair is mandatory.

Having established that the blood supply and nerves are intact, the doctor can begin evaluating the joint or bone afflicted. If there is an obvious deformity, then a fracture or dislocation has occurred. In the absence of obvious deformities, tenderness, redness and swelling may be signs that a fracture has occurred. These signs, however, may occur in many other types of injuries in which there is no bone broken. Consequently, if a fracture is suspected after careful physical examination, x-rays are needed to confirm the diagnosis.

Examining the Neck and Back: [Figure 9B] Neck and back pain are common complaints which the doctor is called upon to evaluate. The same principles that apply to examination of the other joints apply to the examination of the neck and back. The spinal column should be observed and palpated along its entire length. An attempt should

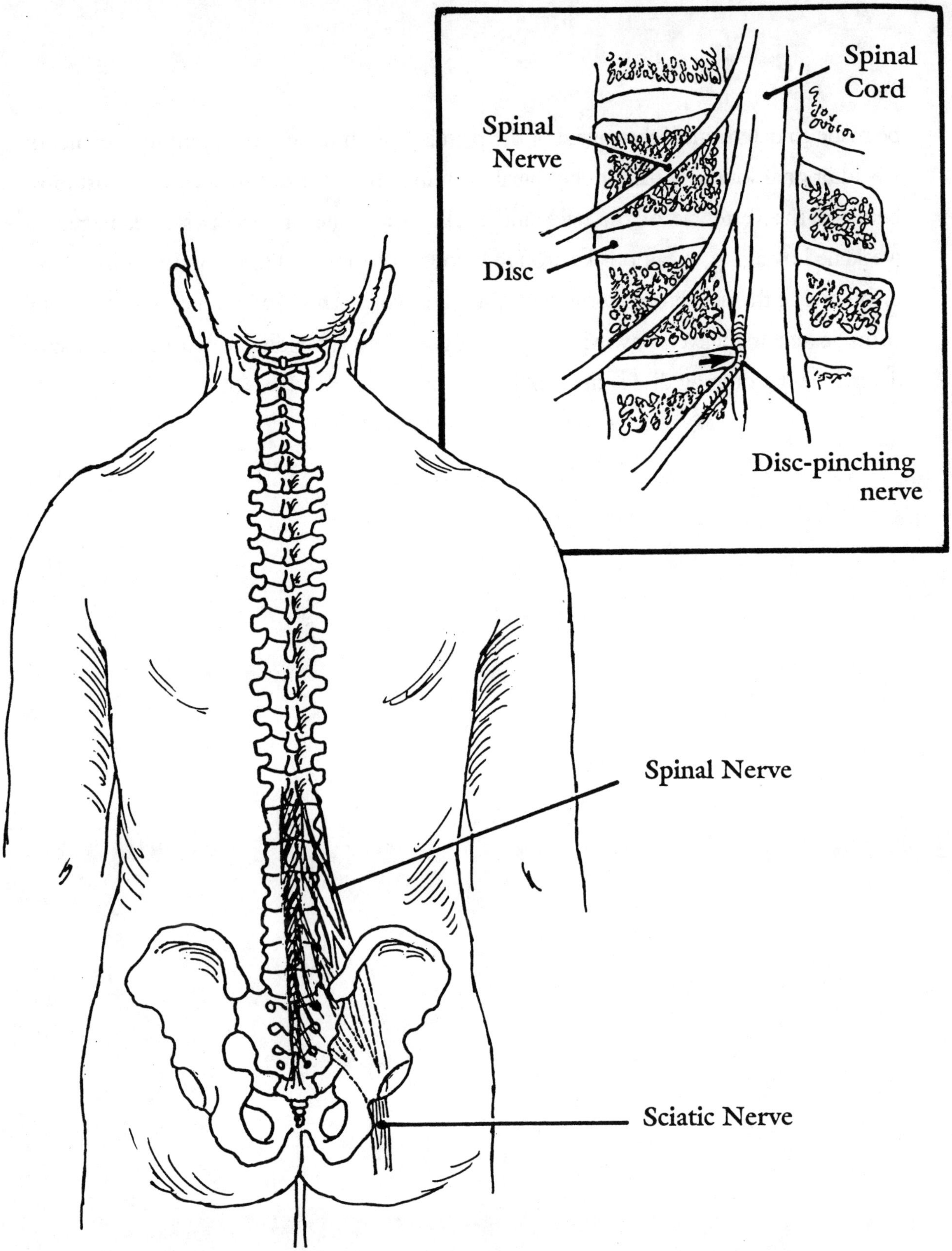

THE VERTEBRAE, SPINE AND PELVIS

Figure 9B

be made to determine if the source of the pain is from muscle, bone, joint or ligaments. An additional source of pain in the spinal column may arise from the discs (or cushions) between the vertebrae of the back and neck. When one of the discs is damaged or weakened by aging, it can break through its outer coating and press on the spinal cord, or on one of the nerve roots coming off the spinal cord. This can be very painful. Several complicated maneuvers involving leg raising and back bending can help the doctor determine if a bulging disc is the problem.

CHAPTER 10

The Male Genitalia

Doctors are aware and sensitive to the fact that patients in general are anxious about the physical examination, particularly as this relates to the examination of a man's genitals. For example, adolescents and men may fear experiencing an erection while being examined. However, such an occurrence is unlikely. In addition, boys and adolescents may worry about whether their genitals are normal. Since there is variation in the size and appearance of the genitals, as there are in all the rest of our body parts, rest assured, in most cases, you're "normal".

Physicians understand these feelings in their patients, and therefore make every effort to examine the genitalia carefully and completely, but also briskly!

The Physical Examination of the male genitalia begins with a visual inspection of the genitals followed by palpation of both the external and internal organs. **[Figure 10A]**

Visual Inspection: During the visual inspection the doctor notes the distribution of pubic hair and the size of the penis and testicles. The secondary sex characteristics are assessed in relationship to the patient's age and general development. The onset of adult development varies from one person to the next. Pubic hair appears and the testicles enlarge between the ages of 12 and 16 years of age. Enlargement of the penis and the ability to ejaculate semen usually occurs between the ages of 13 and 17 years of age.

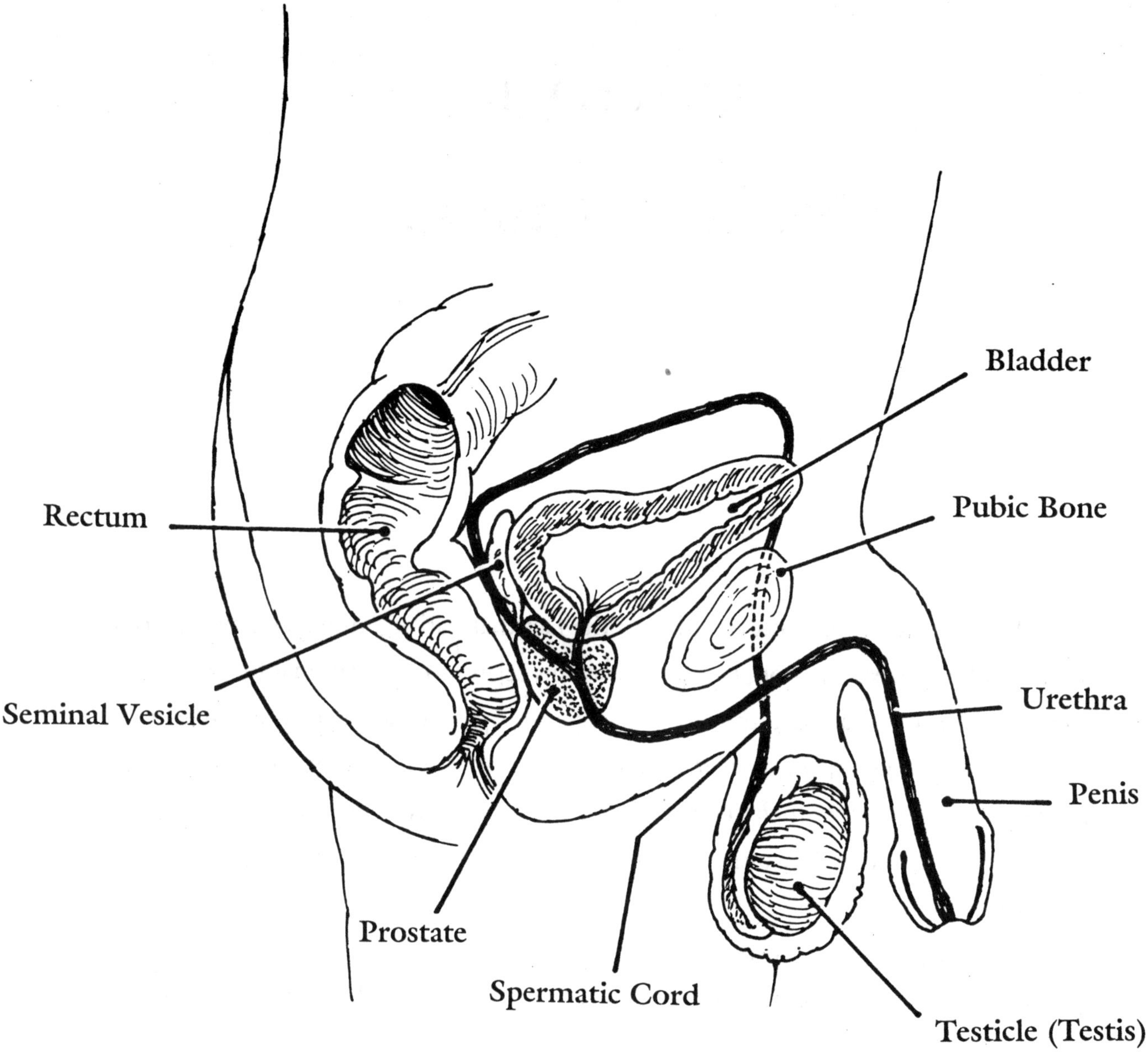

MALE GENITO URINARY SYSTEM

Figure 10A

The Penis: The penis is observed for such things as discharge, the presence of lumps or small knots, wounds or lesions, as well as inflammation and swelling. If the patient is not circumcised, he is asked to retract the foreskin from the head (glans) of the penis so that the glans and foreskin may be observed. The patient is also asked to squeeze the glans so that the doctor may observe the opening at the end tip (meatus) of the penis. If any discharge is observed, a smear is made of the secretion. This is done for the purpose of determining, through culture, the cause of the discharge. If, while taking the history, the patient reports a penile discharge, he is asked to squeeze (milk) the penis from the base to the meatus. If a discharge is present, it is cultured.

The more common penile lesions which are apt to be observed may be syphilitic chancre, condulomata acuminata (venereal warts), and cancer. (The first two listed are sexually transmitted diseases). The syphilitic chancre is the primary lesion of syphilis. It begins as a single pointed pimple that eventually develops into a crater-like ulcer that discharges the germ that causes the disease. As bad as it may appear, it is usually painless. Condylomata acuminata may occur on the glans, foreskin, or shaft of the penis. These growths may either be pink or red in color with a cauliflower-like appearance.

Carcinoma (cancer) of the penis usually appears on the glans and on the inner lip of the foreskin. It may appear dry and scaly, ulcerated, or like a small rounded mass or lump. It is usually painless.

The meatus on most men appears at the end tip of the glans, in the middle. If this opening, however, is on the underside of the glans, but still on the bottom of the glans, the condition is called hypospadias. Urethral openings further back and away from the glans on the underside of the shaft of the penis are referred to as epispadias.

In uncircumcised men it should be easy to pull the foreskin back over the glans of the penis and return it to its original position. Phimosis is a condition in which this is not possible to do. In other words, the foreskin cannot be pulled over the head of the penis. In this situation it is not possible for the doctor to observe the glans or interior surfaces of the foreskin. This condition may also present problems with personal cleanliness. A condition in which the foreskin can be retracted over the glans, but cannot easily be returned to its original position because it tightens around the glans, is called paraphimosis.

Palpation: The shaft of the penis is palpated to determine if there are hard plaque-like structures lodged inside the shaft of the penis in the spongy tissue responsible for erections. The presence of these fibrous structures may make erection painful and penetration during sexual intercourse impossible. This condition is known as Peyronie's Disease.

The Scrotum: With the patient holding his penis out of the way, the doctor is able to visually inspect the scrotum for its general size, appearance and symmetry. The scrotum is naturally more deeply pigmented than the body skin and has a wrinkled appearance. In most men, the left testicle hangs lower than the right one; this is so because the left spermatic cord is generally longer than the right one. Normally, the scrotum hangs loosely from the body; however, influences such as temperature, sexual stimulation, emotional states and age can cause it to move closer up to the body.

Palpation: The scrotum is palpated by spreading out the wrinkled surface of the scrotal sack. This allows for visual inspection to determine if there may be abnormal growths on the scrotum such as sebaceous cysts. (A cyst is a bladder-like sac found in tissue which contains fluid or semi-fluid matter). Sebaceous cysts are firm in texture. They may appear yellow to white in color and are not tender to the touch. These skin lesions may measure up to 1 cm. in diameter.

An unusual thickening of the scrotum caused by an accumulation of fluid in the scrotal sac generally is associated with cardiovascular, kidney or liver disease.

The doctor palpates the testicles using the thumb, index and middle fingers. **[Figure 10B]** The testicles should be sensitive when gently squeezed, but not tender. They should feel smooth and rubbery to the touch, and be free of any bumps or lumps called nodules. In some diseases such as syphilis, a testicle may become completely insensitive to excessive squeezing. Irregularities in the structure or size of the testicles may indicate an infection, cyst or tumor.

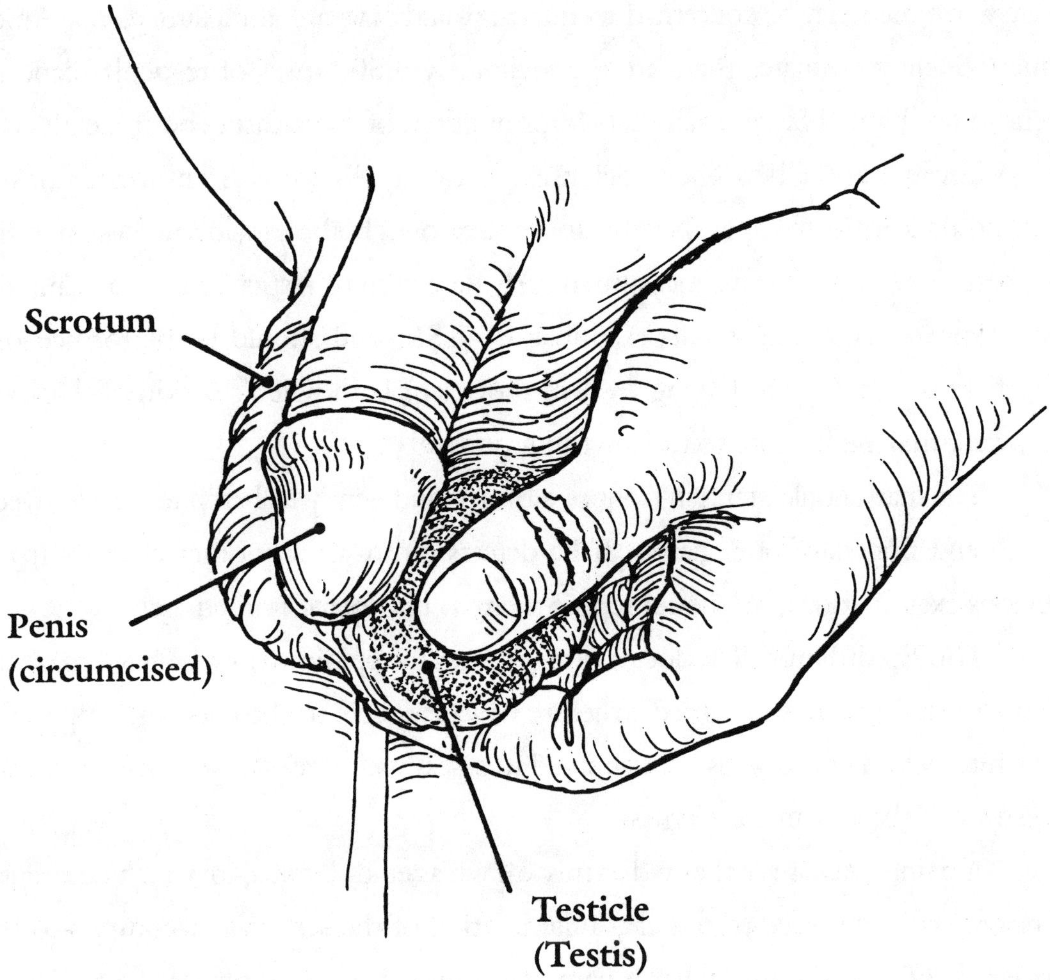

TESTICULAR SELF-EXAMINATION

Figure 10B

Testicular Cancer: While cancer of the testicles is a rare form of cancer, the majority of these cancers occur in young to middle aged men between 20 and 44, a time in life when men may be concerned with fertility and planning for a family. The American Cancer Society estimates there are approximately 5,500 cases of testicular cancer that occur in the United States each year. Four hundred of these cases end in death yearly.

Given that the best line of defense against any disease is an informed consumer, men should learn as much as they can about their own bodies, including how to examine their testicles as a preventive measure in early detection of testicular cancer. This simple test is known as testicular self- examination (TSE) and should be performed once a month. It is best done following a warm shower or bath when the skin of the scrotum is relaxed, making it easier to feel anything unusual.

The man should stand in front of a mirror and gently roll each testicle between his thumb and fingers of both hands. If he detects lumps or any other changes from his previous examinations, he should report them to his doctor immediately.

The Epididymis: The doctor next palpates the epididymis, which is a maze of tiny ducts that make up this C-shaped structure which adheres to the back and upper surface of each testicle. These organs are examined to assess their size, shape, consistency, and to determine if there is any tenderness.

A painful disease of the epididymis known as epididymitis, may include a sensation of heaviness in the affected testicle, inflammation of the scrotum, accompanied by the formation of a small area of hard, painful swelling at the bottom of the testicle. This inflammation is usually associated with a urinary tract infection; however, times of excessive stress may cause these symptoms to appear as well.

The Vas Deferens: The vas deferens are long, thin ducts that come away from each testicle and travel up through the scrotum inside the spermatic cord and up into the abdomen through the inguinal canal. The doctor palpates the vas deferens by grasping each between the thumb and index finger. They should feel like smooth cords that are movable. These structures should not feel beaded or lumpy as the doctor traces them along their path on either side from each testicle to the external inguinal ring, the point at which they enter the abdomen.

Inguinal Hernias: Essentially, a hernia is the protrusion or projection of an organ through the wall of the cavity which normally contains it. Inguinal hernias are conditions in which the inguinal canals serve as passageways for the intestines to protrude through the inguinal canal and into the scrotum. This happens when there is a weakness in the abdominal muscles that separate the abdomen from the inguinal canals.

The inguinal canals are the passageway through which the spermatic cords pass from the abdomen into the scrotum. It is this passageway that the testicles follow in descending from the abdominal cavity (where they develop embryonically) into the scrotum just before birth. One and one half inches in length, they have an internal opening where they meet the abdomen called the internal ring. The other end that opens into the scrotum is called the external ring.

There are two types of inguinal hernias: direct and indirect.

a) Direct Inguinal Hernias: The doctor examines for direct inguinal hernias by placing two fingers over each external ring and instructing the patient to bear down as if having a bowel movement. The presence of a direct hernia will produce a bulge that the doctor can feel.

b) Indirect Hernias: The hernia is indirect if it lies up inside the inguinal canal. To determine the presence of an indirect hernia, the doctor inserts a finger into the path of the inguinal canal. **[Figure 10C]** When the finger passes as far as it will go, the patient is asked to turn his head (so he won't cough on the doctor) and cough. A hernia, if present, will be felt as a mass of tissue meeting the finger and then withdrawing. In cases of extreme weakening of the abdominal musculature, the intestine may pass all the way through the inguinal canal and into the scrotum. Indirect hernias occur more frequently in young men and are the most common of the abdominal hernias.

Examination of the Anus, Rectum and Prostate: While it is recognized that the rectal examination is generally uncomfortable and embarrassing for the patient, it provides such

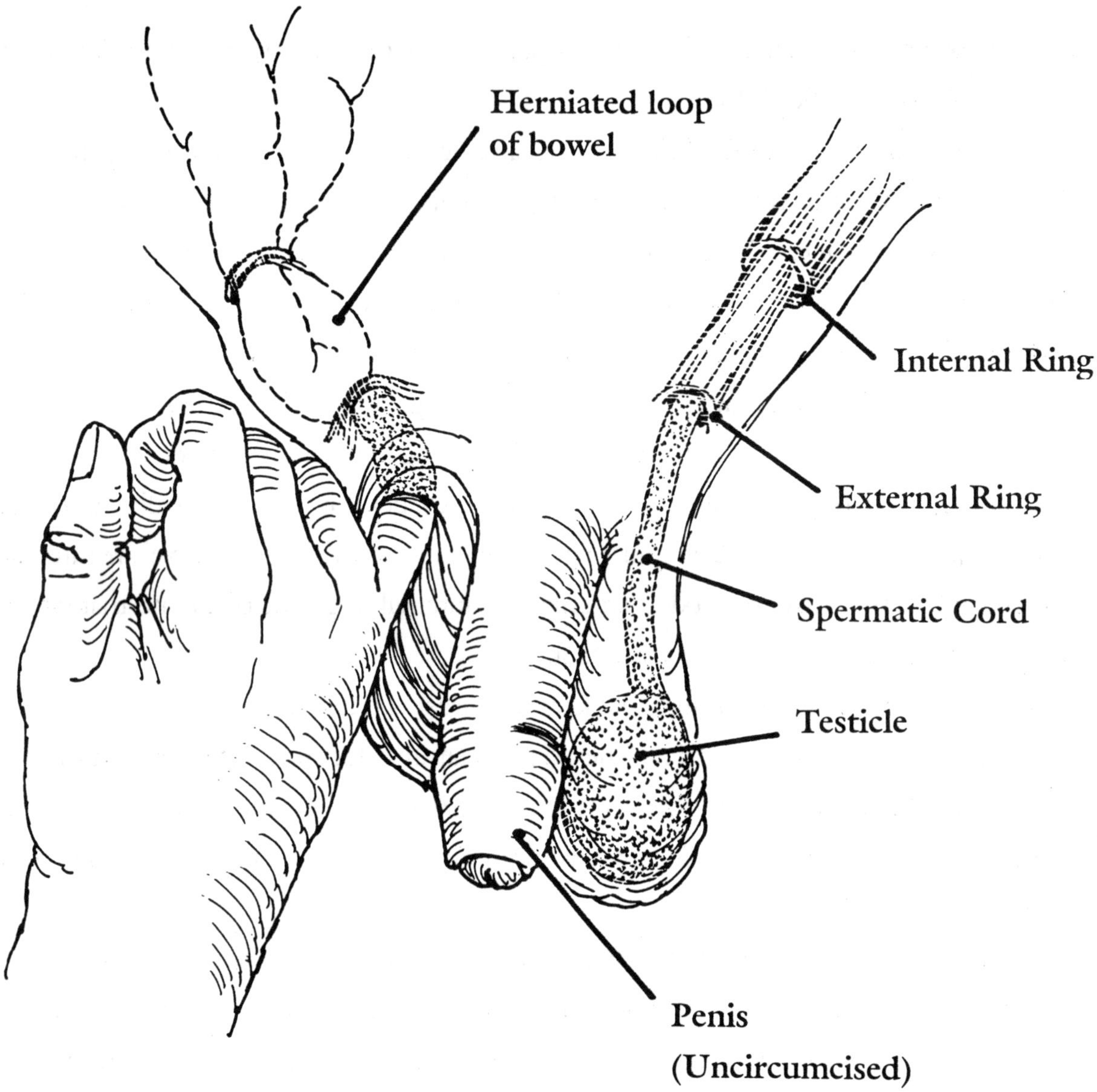

EXAMINATION OF INDIRECT HERNIA

Figure 10C

important information that it cannot be overlooked as part of a comprehensive and thorough examination of the body.

Visual Examination: The first thing the doctor does in visually inspecting the anal region is to look for the presence of lumps, rashes and inflammations. In carefully inspecting the anus itself, the doctor looks for skin lesions, warts and external hemorrhoids.

Palpation of the Anus, Rectum and Prostate: This examination is done with the patient standing, hips flexed, with his upper body bent over, supported by the examining table.

Carefully placing the pad of the index finger over the anal opening, the doctor gently pushes the finger into the rectum. The patient is asked to bear down to relax the anal muscles. As relaxation occurs, the tip of the finger more easily enters the anal canal. The patient is warned that there may be a feeling of urgency for a bowel movement. The doctor rotates the finger to examine the muscular structures within. Inserting the finger still further, the doctor feels for any irregularities like tenderness, lumps, masses of tissue, polyps or internal hemorrhoids. The walls of the rectum should feel smooth and even. The doctor next palpates the prostate gland. **[Figure 10D]** Feeling this organ may make the patient feel like he wants to urinate, but he will not. The doctor notes the size, contour, consistency and the mobility of the prostate gland. The gland should feel like a pencil eraser -- firm, smooth, and slightly movable. It should not be tender. Any deviations from the normal size, shape and consistency of the prostate gland may be indicative of enlargement of the gland, which may lead to difficulties in urinating. The presence of lumps or a change in its consistency may indicate cancer.

The Prostate Gland: The prostate gland is a structure about the size and shape of a chestnut. Anatomically, it is located at the base of the bladder. The urethra, the tube that conveys urine from the bladder through the penis to the outside, passes through the prostate gland.

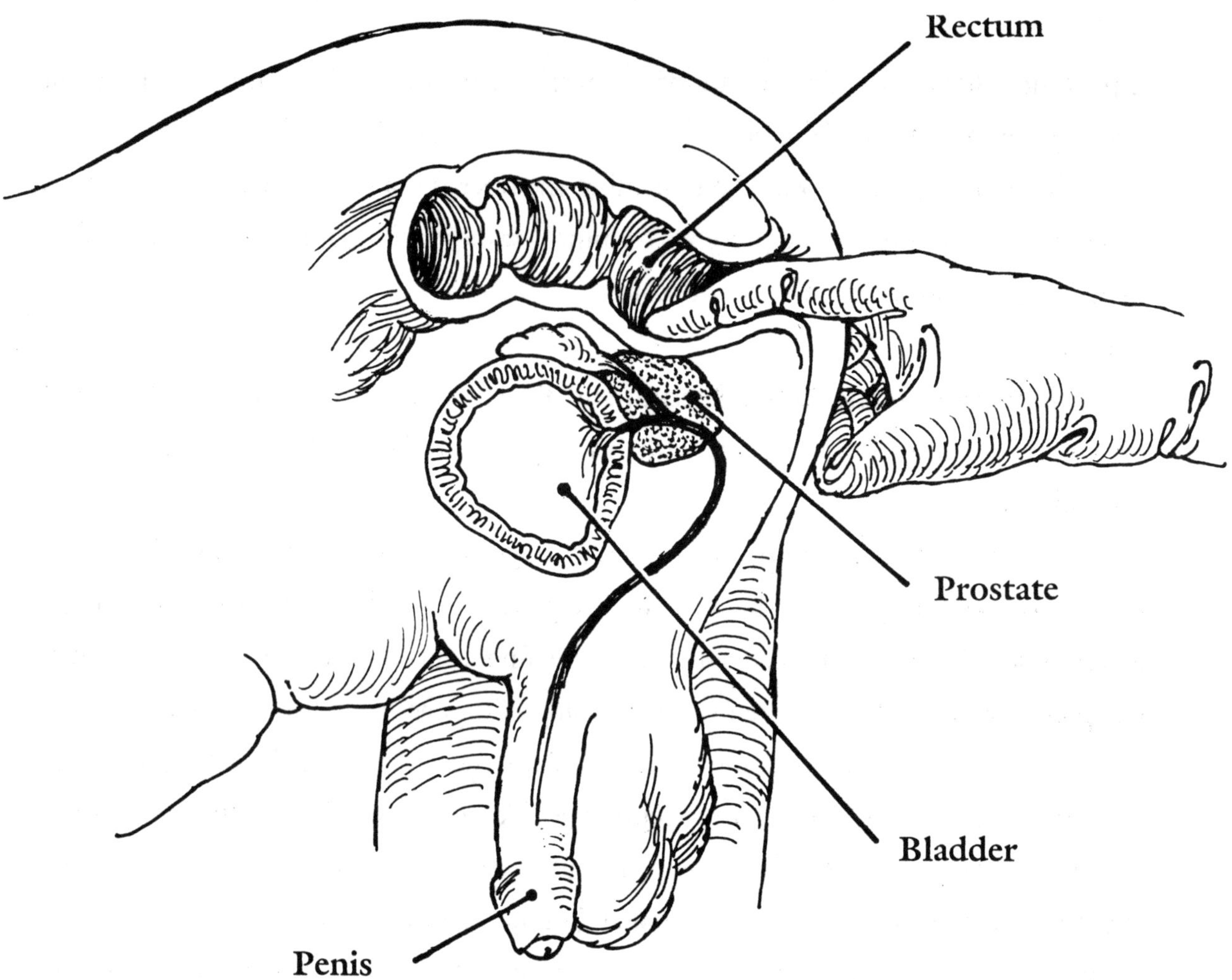

EXAMINATION OF THE PROSTATE

Figure 10D

During sexual excitement, sperms move into the prostate gland and mix with various secretions produced by the prostate gland and seminal vesicles to make up semen. At the time of ejaculation, the prostate gland contracts, ejecting the semen through the urethra. Thus the prostate gland plays a significant and important role in a man's sexuality. Like all organs of the human body, it too is subjected to various infections and diseases.

Among some of the more common ailments of the prostate gland are prostatis and cancer.

Prostatitis, a condition in which the prostate gland becomes enlarged and inflamed, usually as a result of various infectious agents (like those responsible for sexually transmitted diseases). This condition may occur in men of any age. Symptoms may include difficulty in urinating, feelings of urgency to urinate frequently, a burning sensation while urinating, bloody semen, cloudy penile discharge, aching testicles, pain in the pelvic area or base of the penis, back ache, lower abdominal ache, and difficulties with sexual functions, like painful erections or ejaculations.

Cancer of the Prostate Gland: According to the American Cancer Society, approximately 22,000 men die from this form of cancer each year. As with most cancers, early detection can provide early diagnosis and treatment. Consequently, it is important for men to know and be aware of the signs and symptoms of this disease, which may include many of those already listed above for prostatitis. Men should also be sensitive to weak or interrupted flow of urine, inability to urinate, or the presence of blood in the urine. Persistent low back pain, or pain in the upper thighs and pelvic area should also be reported to a doctor. Since the potential for developing this form of cancer becomes greater with increasing age, an annual rectal examination for men over 40 years of age is highly recommended.

CHAPTER 11

The Gynecological Exam

Gynecology is the study of human femaleness. A gynecologist is a physician who cares for and treats women with a focus on reproduction and the reproductive organs. A related field is obstetrics, the study of women and childbirth. An obstetrician is a physician concerned with caring for and treating women in connection with childbirth. Doctors who specialize in the female reproductive area train in both gynecology and obstetrics.

Many women are apprehensive about having a gynecological exam. The exam can make the patient feel exposed, vulnerable and embarrassed. However, doctors are taught gentle and compassionate skills to make the exam the best possible experience for the patient. These skills include conducting the examination in a sensitive but straightforward manner. This involves listening to the patient attentively and answering questions she may have, explaining the procedures to her, and educating the woman about her body (this may include letting the woman view the pelvic examination with a mirror whenever deemed appropriate). Women should take active steps to learn about their bodies and enter into a partnership with their gynecologist, where both assume responsibility for the woman's health.

The Gynecological Examination:

A gynecological examination is performed on a woman with the focus on evaluation of her reproductive organs. Doctors encourage women to have a gynecological exam each year beyond the age of 18 and for the rest of their lives. One reason for this is that a complete gynecological exam can detect more than half of all cancers that affect women today. These are cancers of the breast, cervix, ovary, bladder, rectum, endometrium and vulva.

A woman should have her first gynecological exam around the age of 18 or when she becomes sexually active, whichever comes first. The time when a girl has her first menstrual period, usually occurring between the ages of 11-17, is called menarche. The time when a woman stops having menstrual periods is called menopause and occurs between the ages of 45-50. Although it is an important examination for any woman, the gynecological exam is *most* important for women who are sexually active.

The gynecological exam consists of two parts: the patient's history and the physical examination. While obtaining a history, a physician may ask specific questions concerning previous pregnancies, contraception and past gynecological history. The physical should include a total examination with special attention paid to the breasts and reproductive organs by pelvic examination.

Examination of the Breasts:

First, the breasts are inspected by the physician while the patient is sitting upright. The appearance and texture of the breasts are evaluated in this part of the examination. With the patient's arms at her sides, the physician looks for changes in the appearance of the patient's breasts, noting bumps, flattenings, or unequal shapes. Any change in breast appearance may be indicative of an underlying tumor. Tumors can be cancerous (malignant) or non-cancerous (benign). Next, the nipples are examined. A deviated (or crooked) nipple may indicate a tumor growing underneath it that is forcing the skin to pull it from its normal shape. Tumors come in many different sizes and irregular shapes.

Following observation of the breasts, the physician thoroughly palpates (or feels) the breasts. Palpation is performed with the patient lying on her back with her hands behind her head. Palpation is carried out to note any changes in the way the breasts feel from the previous exam. A lump, an area of thickening, or an area of tenderness are all things that can be discovered upon palpation. The physician also checks the nipples for any discharge by gently squeezing them. A breast discharge may be indicative of cancer, infection, or other problems. If the patient does not know how to perform breast self-examination, the physician should instruct the patient how to do so. **[Figures 11A, 11B]**

Mammography:

Mammography is the use of X-rays to examine the breasts. This procedure is invaluable because it can detect a tumor before there are any clinical signs and symptoms and before there has been time for cancer cells to spread to other parts of the body. Once a malignant tumor has had time to spread, it is difficult to completely cure the patient of cancer. Early detection of a (malignant) tumor through mammography can offer treatment early on and cure the patient of cancer 90% of the time. Malignant tumors are treated with chemotherapy, radiation, or surgery, depending on the size and extent of spread. Experts disagree on when women should have their first mammograms. Usually, routine mammograms are not recommended before the age of 40.

The External Pelvic Exam:

The pelvic exam is carried out gently by the physician. **[Figure 11C]** The doctor inspects and palpates the lower abdomen. The physician is looking for any enlargements, tenderness, masses, hernias (protrusions under the skin) or incisions. The amount of pubic, facial, and underarm hair and its distribution is also noted. A small or large amount of hair can be an indicator of a hormonal imbalance.

The pelvic exam is performed with the woman lying on her back on a special table with stirrups (foot holders) at one end. She is placed in the lithotomy position which means that her heels are placed in the stirrups with her buttocks extending past the end

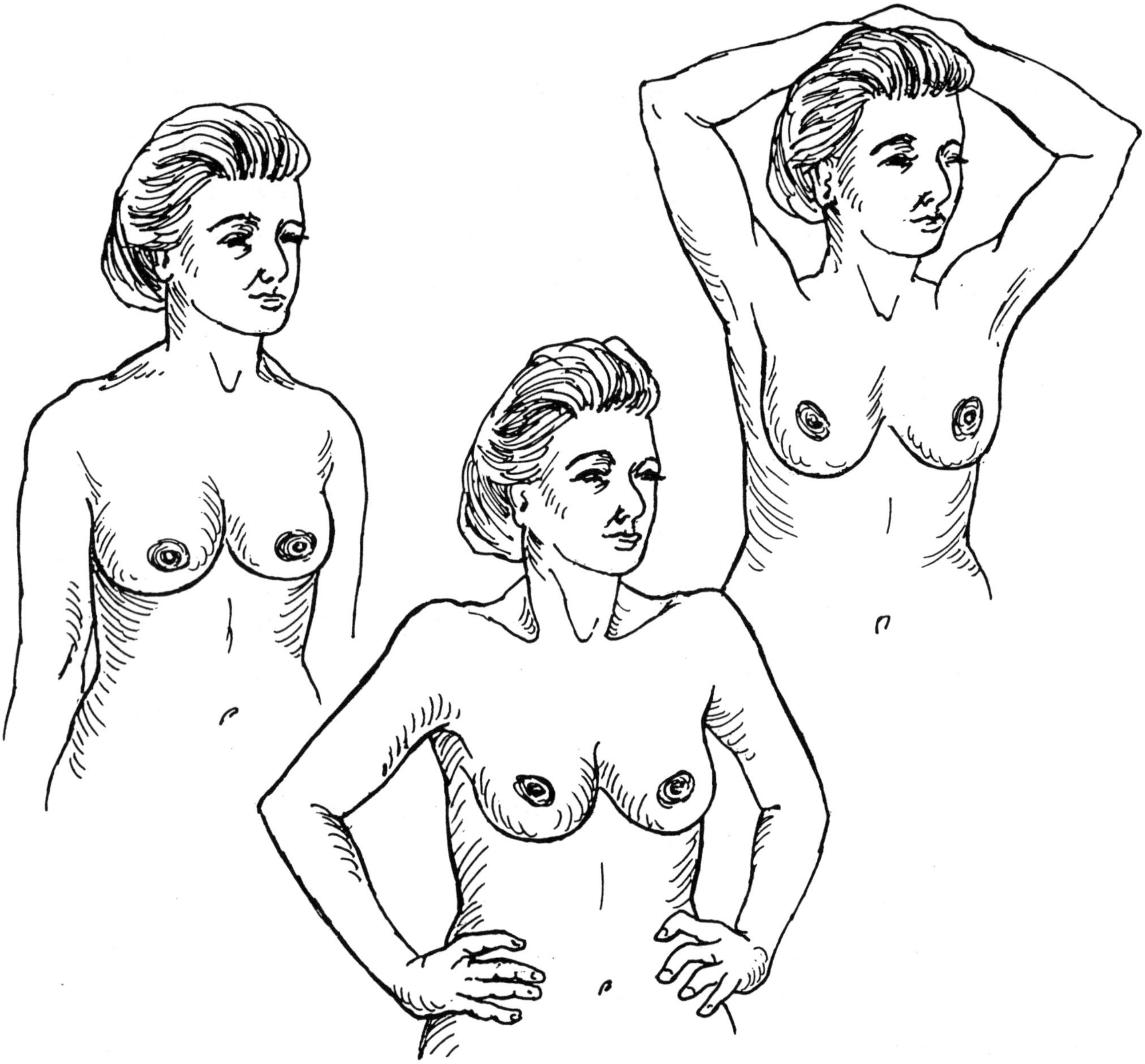

BREAST SELF EXAM -- OBSERVATION

Figure 11A

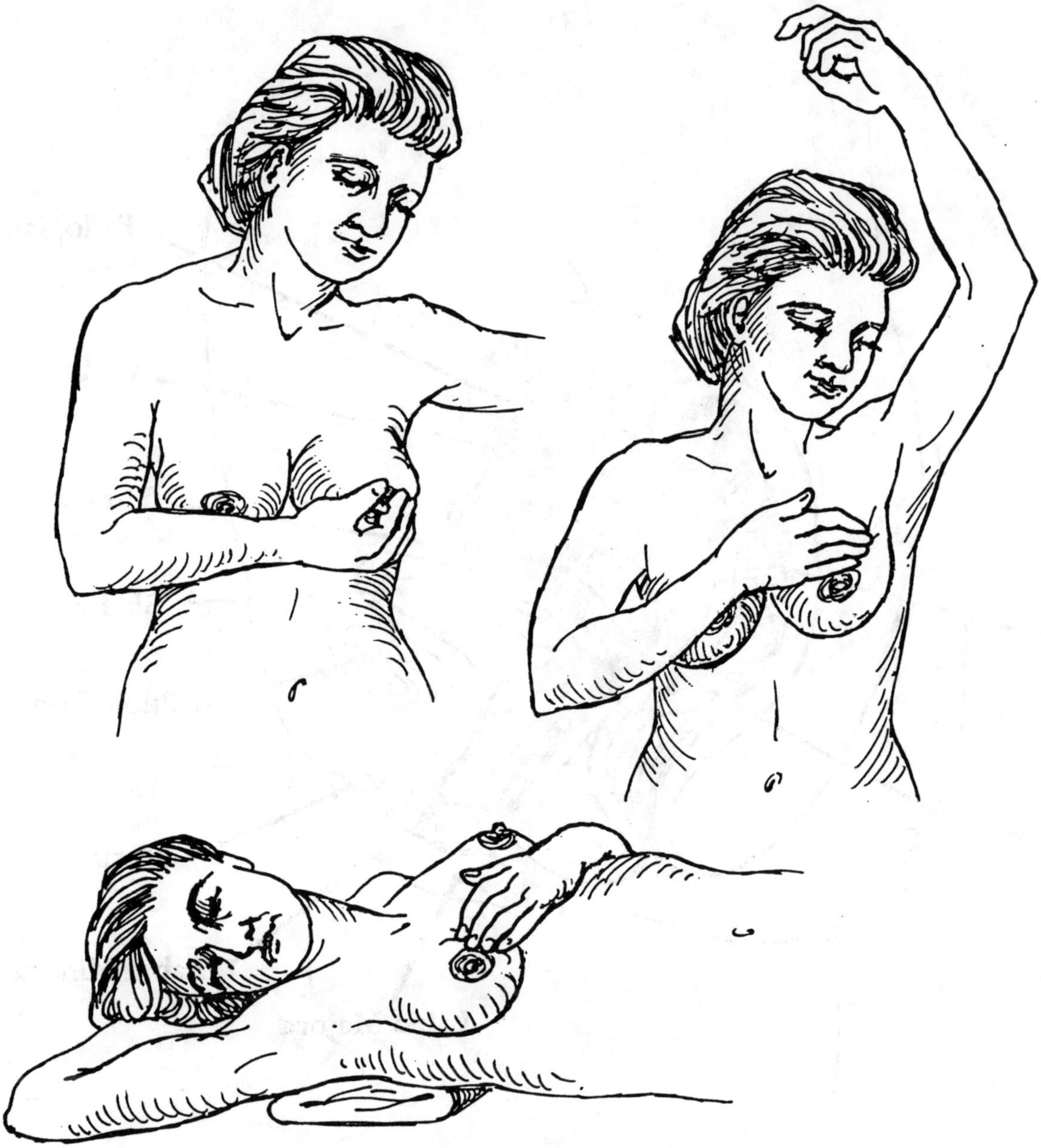

BREAST SELF EXAM -- PALPATION

Figure 11B

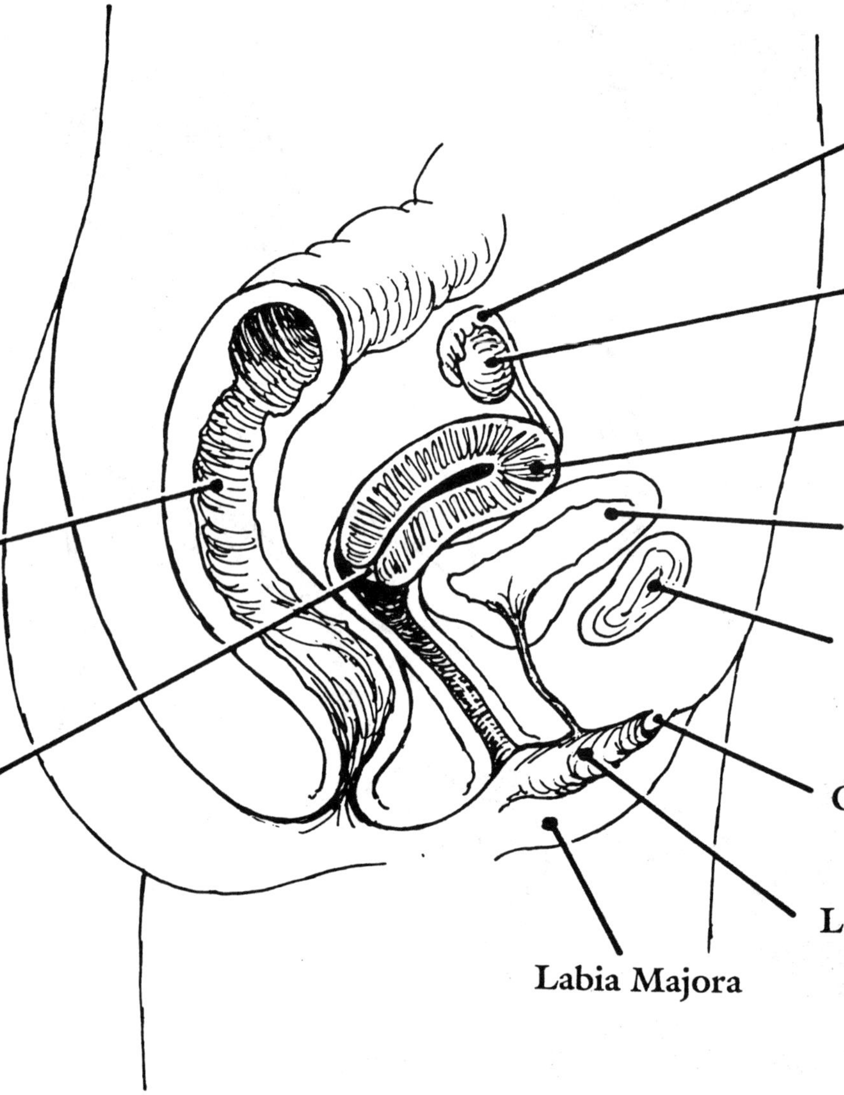

FEMALE GENITO URINARY SYSTEM

Figure 11C

of the table. This position relaxes the abdominal muscles and straightens the lower region of the spine (called the lumbar region).

The external genitalia are next inspected and palpated. **[Figure 11D]** This external portion of a woman's genitals are collectively referred to as the vulva. This area is carefully examined for warts, irritation, tumors, scarring or sores. Next, the labia minora and labia majora are separated to examine the hymen, urethral opening and opening to the vagina. The size of the clitoris and the development of the labia minora and majora are also noted.

The Internal Pelvic Exam:

The internal examination begins with the insertion of an instrument called the speculum into the vagina which is used to separate and hold apart the walls of the vagina. **[Figures 11E and 11F]** When inserting the speculum, the physician makes sure it is warm and lubricated with water. With a bright light aiding the physician's sight, the cervix (entrance to the uterus) is inspected. The area is examined for ulcerations, cysts, bleeding, enlargements or menstrual discharge. The positioning of the cervix is also noted. For instance, if the cervix points toward the bladder, then the uterus will be bent backward and will point toward the lower spinal chord or sacrum. This condition is called retroversion.

The Pap Test:

This test, named after Dr. George Papanicolaou, is good for detecting early stages in the development of cervical cancers. With the speculum in place, the doctor gently scrapes some cells from the cervix and vagina with a swab. These cells are examined for the purpose of detecting cancerous cells. Cancerous and precancerous cells appear different from normal cells. This test for early detection of cancer has been very useful in reducing the death rate due to cancer of the cervix by 50 percent.

Following the pap test the speculum is removed slowly while the physician inspects the vaginal walls for vaginitis (inflammation of the vagina), discharges, cysts,

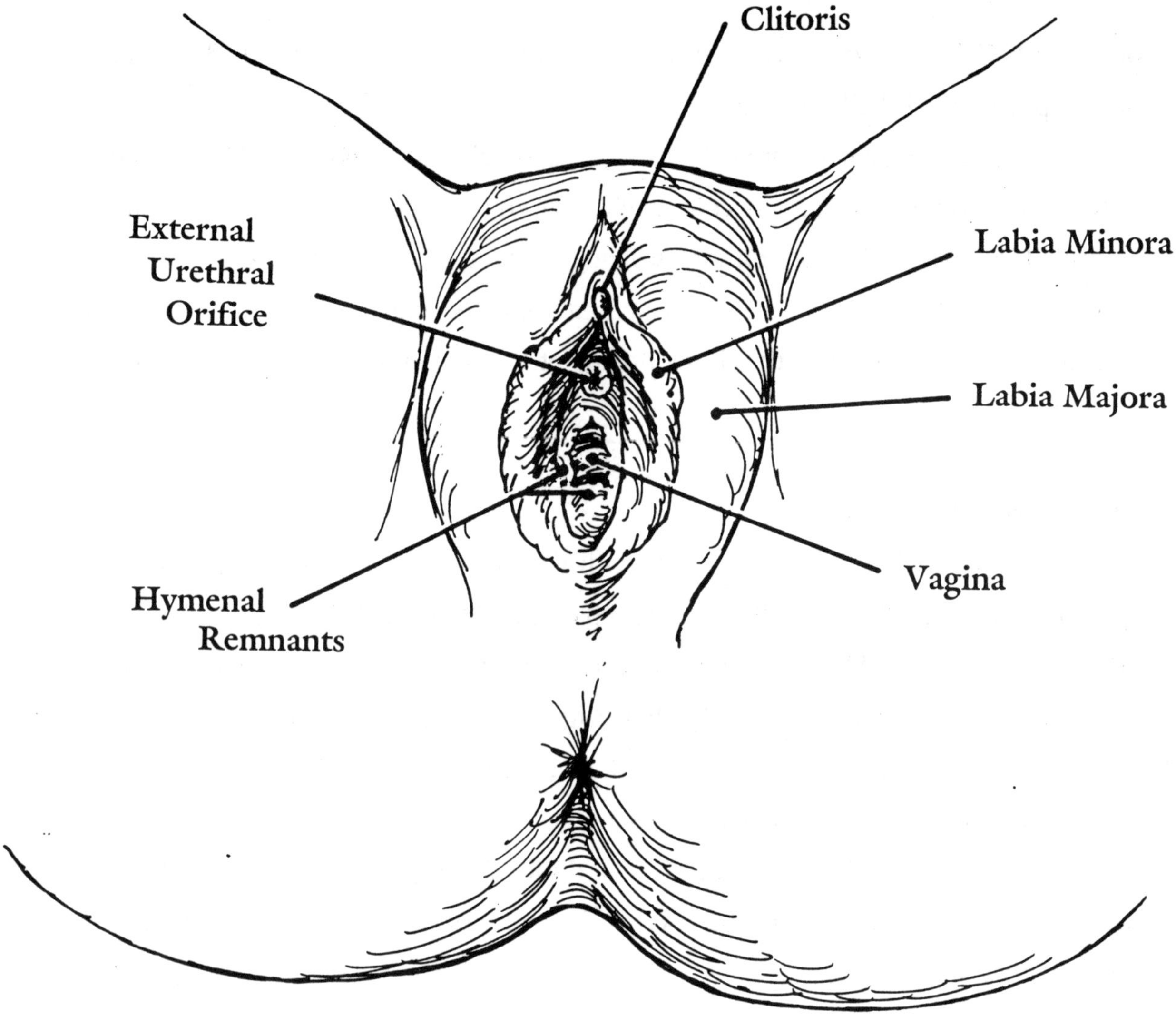

FEMALE EXTERNAL GENITALIA

Figure 11D

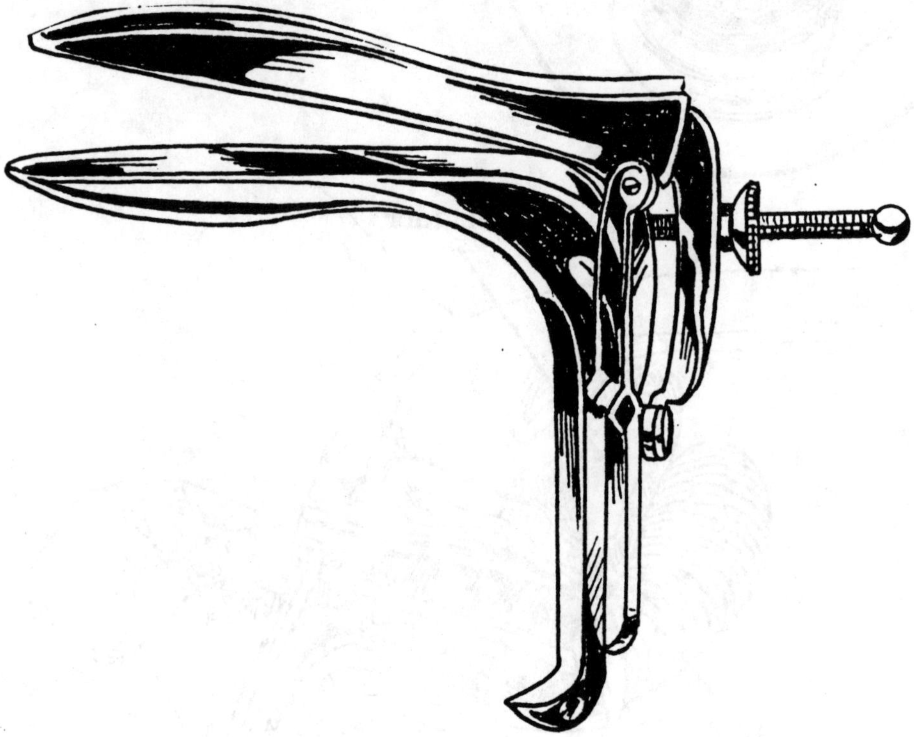

THE SPECULUM

Figure 11E

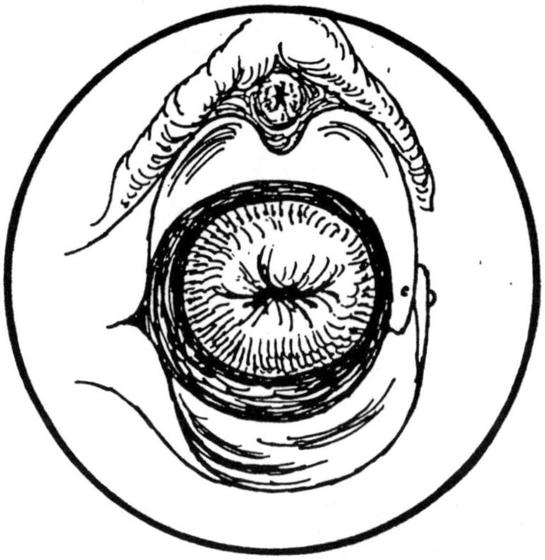

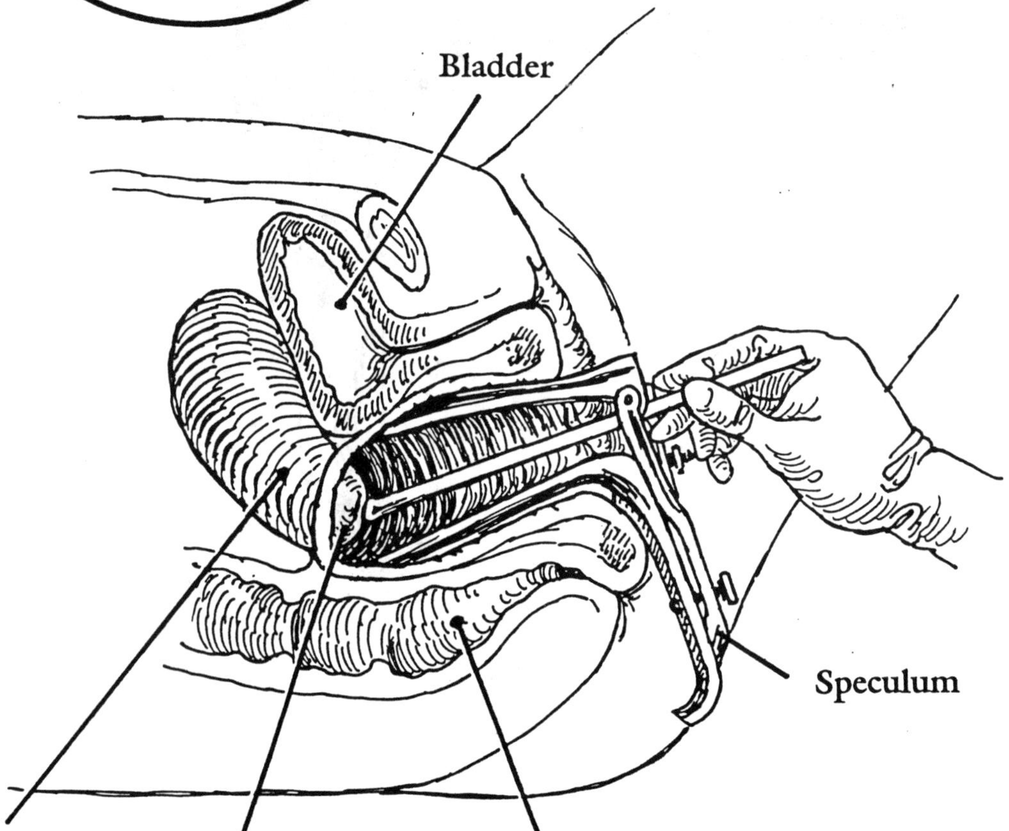

INTERNAL EXAMINATION WITH SPECULUM

Figure 11F

or other lesions that may have been missed because of the presence of the speculum. Other cervical or vaginal tests may be conducted during the exam, such as obtaining a specimen of a discharge to determine the cause of an infection.

The Bimanual Examination:

Using both hands for this procedure the doctor is able to examine the cervix, uterus, ovaries, fallopian tubes and bladder. With the index and middle fingers of the left hand inserted into the vagina and the other hand placed on the abdomen, the doctor first identifies the cervix and then the uterus. **[Figure 11G]** The uterus is ordinarily pear-shaped, firm, smooth, moveable and not tender. The physician now tries to identify the ovaries and fallopian tubes. The normal fallopian tube cannot be felt as a distinct structure and the woman may feel a bit of pain as it is being palpated. The ovaries are more easily palpated, although in heavier patients it may be more difficult. The entire region is felt for masses and tenderness. If a mass is felt, its characteristics and location are carefully noted. The bimanual exam also includes palpation of the bladder. Again the doctor feels for abnormal shape, masses, or tenderness.

The Rectovaginal Exam:

With the index finger in the vagina and the middle finger in the rectum, the physician can feel more accurately the posterior surface of the uterus, cervical ligaments (tough bands of tissue that hold the cervix in place), the ovaries and the side walls of the pelvis. The shape of the rectum is noted as the physician removes the finger. Feces that adhere to the gloves are examined for mucous or blood. Thus, this procedure may also detect rectal disorders. The pelvic examination should be gentle and careful. Tightened and anxious muscles make the examination unnecessarily uncomfortable. A woman who can relax while she is examined is likely to find that the whole experience was not as uncomfortable as she might have anticipated.

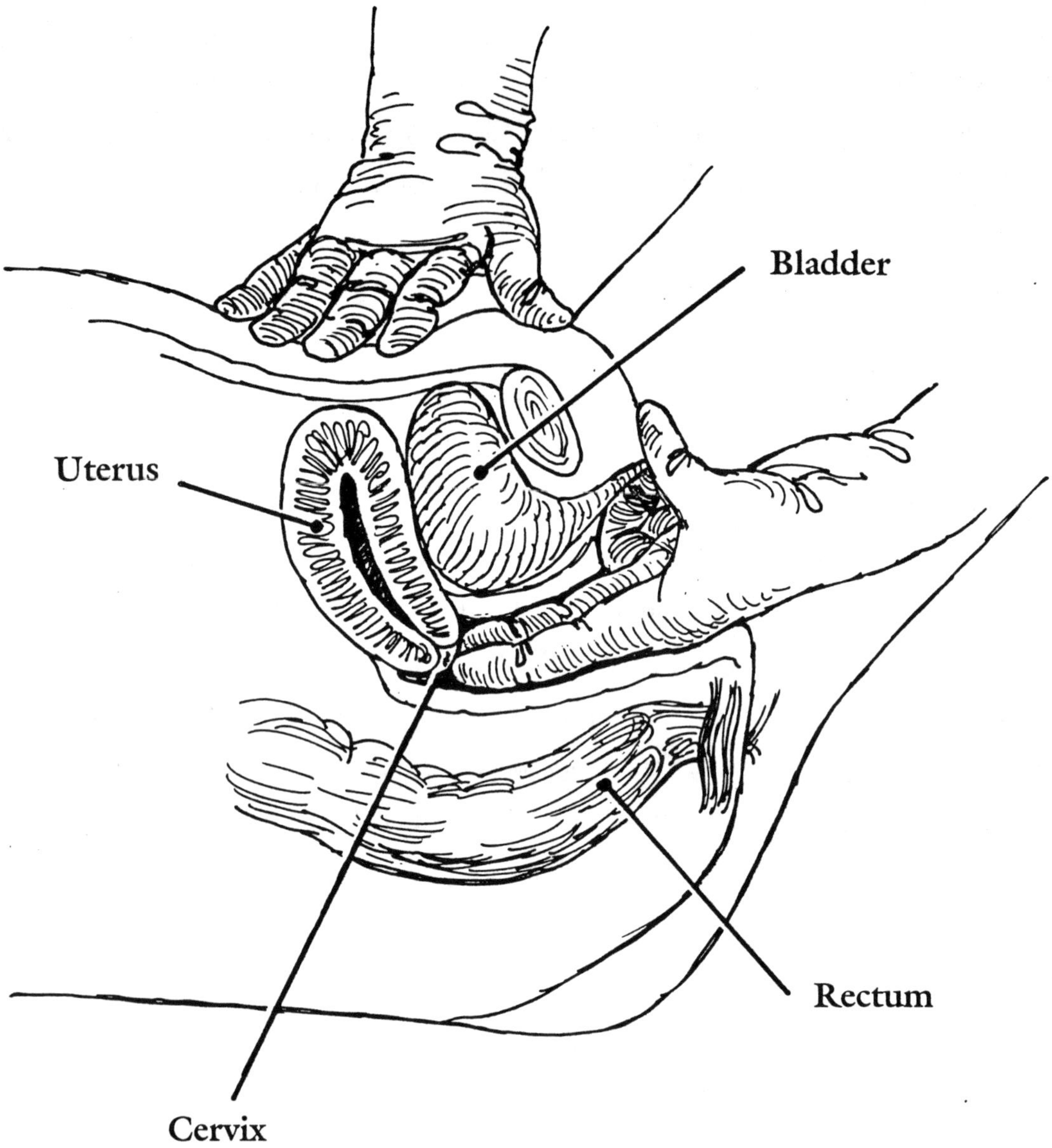

BI-MANUAL PELVIC EXAMINATION

Figure 11G

CHAPTER 12

The Nervous system

The nervous system is the most complex system of the human body. It is generally considered by doctors to be the most difficult to understand, examine, diagnose and treat. Because of its complexity, it is the most poorly understood system and one of the most difficult to explain. Despite the relatively little that is known about the nervous system, the knowledge that is available to medical science could fill several medical encyclopedias.

The brain is the central control center of all the functions of the body **(See Figure 12A)**. Without your even thinking about it, the brain controls your rate of breathing, blood pressure, body temperature and hundreds of other unconscious processes such as digestion of food and elimination of waste.

Divisions of the Brain:

The brain, while clearly the most complex electrical wiring system ever designed, is often subdivided in several ways for simplicity. For example, the left and right sides, the sympathetic and parasympathetic systems, and higher and lower areas, are distinguished. The higher areas are further divided into localized areas which have specific functions. These divisions will be discussed briefly. It may help to refer to Figure 12A as you read.

1. Right and left sides: Generally, the right side of the brain controls the left side of the body, and vice versa. There are connections between the two sides of the brain which allow for coordination of the left and right sides of the body. In addition,

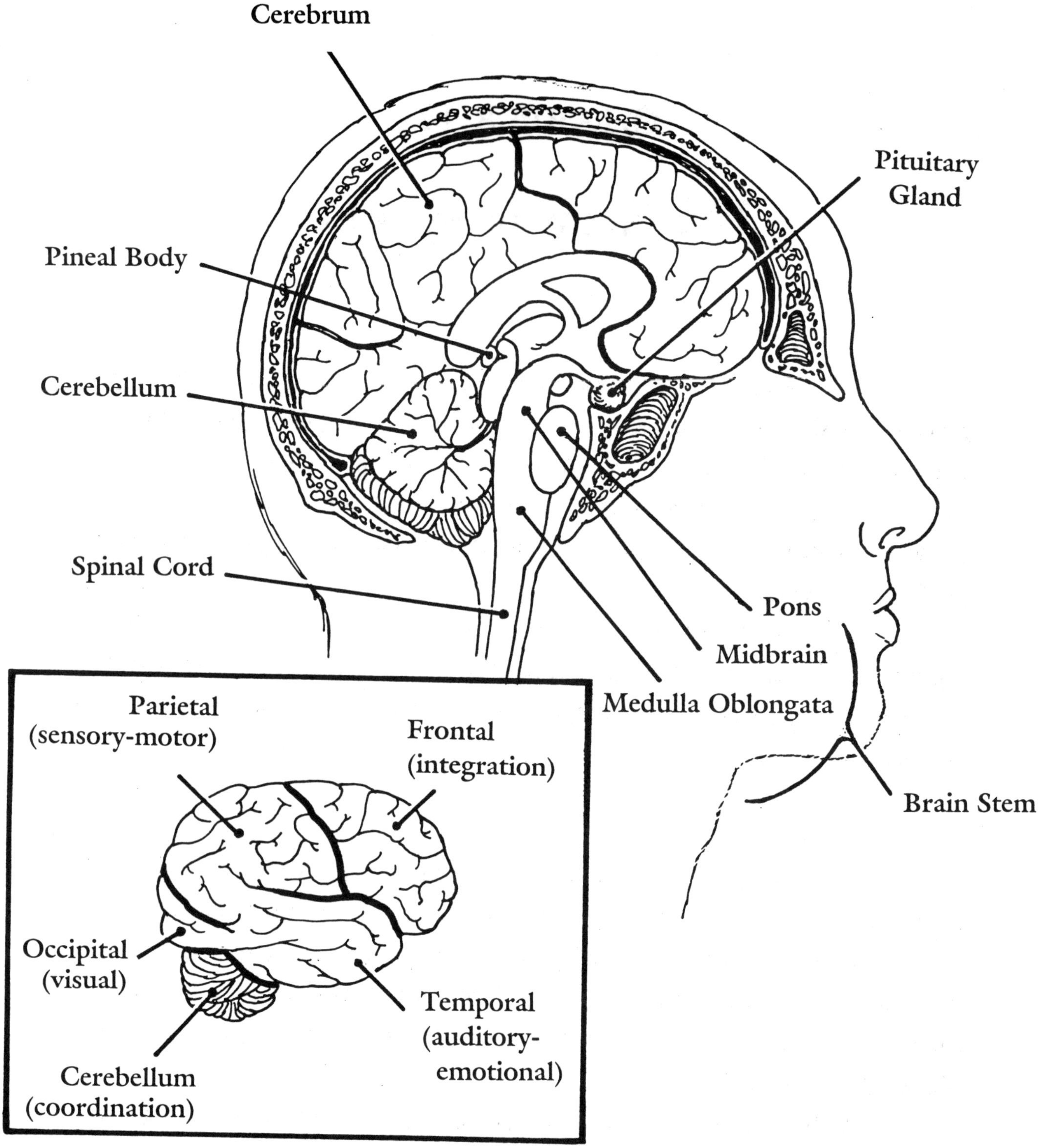

THE BRAIN

Figure 12A

the left side of the brain, in most people, stores and executes language functions, while the right side usually controls creative and artistic thought.

2. Sympathetic and parasympathetic systems: The sympathetic system, in essence, speeds up bodily functions. When activated, it increases heart rate, respirations, and dilates the pupils (among other things). It is activated in situations of fear or pain. The parasympathetic system works the opposite way and does things like slow the heart rate and respirations. These two systems are never completely "on" or "off" but always attempt to balance each other to maintain the body at a steady state under normal conditions.

3. Higher and lower divisions: The more complex a function is, the higher in the brain it is controlled. For example, mathematic calculations occur in the cerebrum which is the most complex (highest) part of the brain. The more simple functions, which are generally automatic and reflexive, are controlled from lower brain centers. An example here would be the breathing center which is located in the brain stem. The simplest functions are controlled at the level of the spinal cord, as in the case of the knee-jerk reflex.

4. Finally, the cerebrum is divided into areas with specific functions: The frontal areas integrate complex thoughts and ideas and affect personality, while the temporal areas sense and interpret sound and control emotions. The occipital areas receive and interpret visual information from the eyes, while the parietal areas interpret sensation and motor (muscle) output.

Examination of the Nervous System:

The goal of examining the nervous system is to see if there are any neurological problems which could signal disease. Because the various nerve cells in the brain are arranged into specialized areas, and because they are interconnected in specific ways, a doctor can use the information obtained in a neurological exam to determine where in the nervous system a certain abnormality may be located. So, doing a neurological exam on a patient who complains of weakness, dizziness, or loss of muscle function is much like a detective searching for clues. The answers found by the doctor enable him or her to predict where in the nervous system the problem is located. For example, if a patient complains of weakness in the hand, the problem could be in the nerves which run down the arm, or in the spinal cord, or in the lower or upper part of the brain. By doing a careful neurological exam the doctor should be able to assemble all the findings (clues) and determine where in the nervous system the problem originates.

Most doctors divide their examination of the nervous system into three parts: 1) the examination of the patient's mental status and level of consciousness; 2) the examination of the nerves in the head; and, 3) the examination of the nerves in the rest of the body.

1. Mental Status and Level of Consciousness

The first step in examining the nervous system is ascertaining the level of consciousness of the patient. Are they awake and alert or are they sleepy, lethargic, obtunded (almost unresponsive), or even comatose (not responsive at all)? If a patient is not awake and alert, this could be an important clue to many potentially serious conditions such as a brain tumor, meningitis (infection of the membrane around the brain), head injury, stroke, or metabolic imbalances in the body.

The second step is making sure that the higher functions of the brain are intact. These would include such complex functions as memory, speech, personal identity, and a general orientation to the situation at hand. To test these functions doctors ask several simple questions: What is your name?, Where are we now?, What is today's date?, and Why are you here? A patient who can answer all of these correctly is said to be fully oriented. A person who has difficulty with one or more of these questions may have had a brain injury or may have an underlying problem with higher brain functions such as mental retardation or dementia.

2. Nerves in the Head (Cranial Nerves)

There are twelve pairs of cranial nerves. The nerves which branch out directly from under the brain are called cranial nerves. They control most functions of the head and some in the neck and lower body organs. Doctors frequently examine cranial nerves with simple tests to determine that they are all intact and functioning correctly.

The functions of the twelve pairs of cranial nerves are diverse. They receive complex input signals from the senses and provide output signals which control a myriad of body functions. The cranial nerves are responsible for sensing five sensory inputs: smell, taste, sight, sound, and touch. The cranial nerves also control movements like chewing, eye focussing, swallowing, and gagging. They also control very complicated reflexes such as the reflex that makes you blink your eyes when dangerous objects are approaching. Doctors have both simple and complex ways of testing each pair of cranial nerves. The tests doctors do when examining the cranial nerves enable them to determine where the problem is in the nerves or brain. Also, the tests help them diagnose the disease which is involved. For a more detailed description of how doctors examine the cranial nerves, see the Appendix.

3. Nerves in the Body (spinal nerves):

At the base of the brain, a large collection of nerve cells leaves the skull together, forming the spinal cord. It is through the spinal cord that most of the body's sensory information from the body (input) travels to the brain. The spinal cord also carries the nerves for motor commands (movement of muscles) from the brain to the rest of the body (output).

The spinal cord is the conduit through which the entire body is controlled from the neck down. **[Figure 12B]** Exiting from the spinal cord are 31 pairs of nerves. They leave the spinal cord at different levels all the way from the neck to the tailbone. The structure of the spinal cord is arranged in a manner that allows for disease or injury of a specific part of it to produce predictable neurological symptoms. It is the doctor's job, by examining the patient's body, to correlate the symptoms with physical findings and thus diagnose the disease process responsible for a problem.

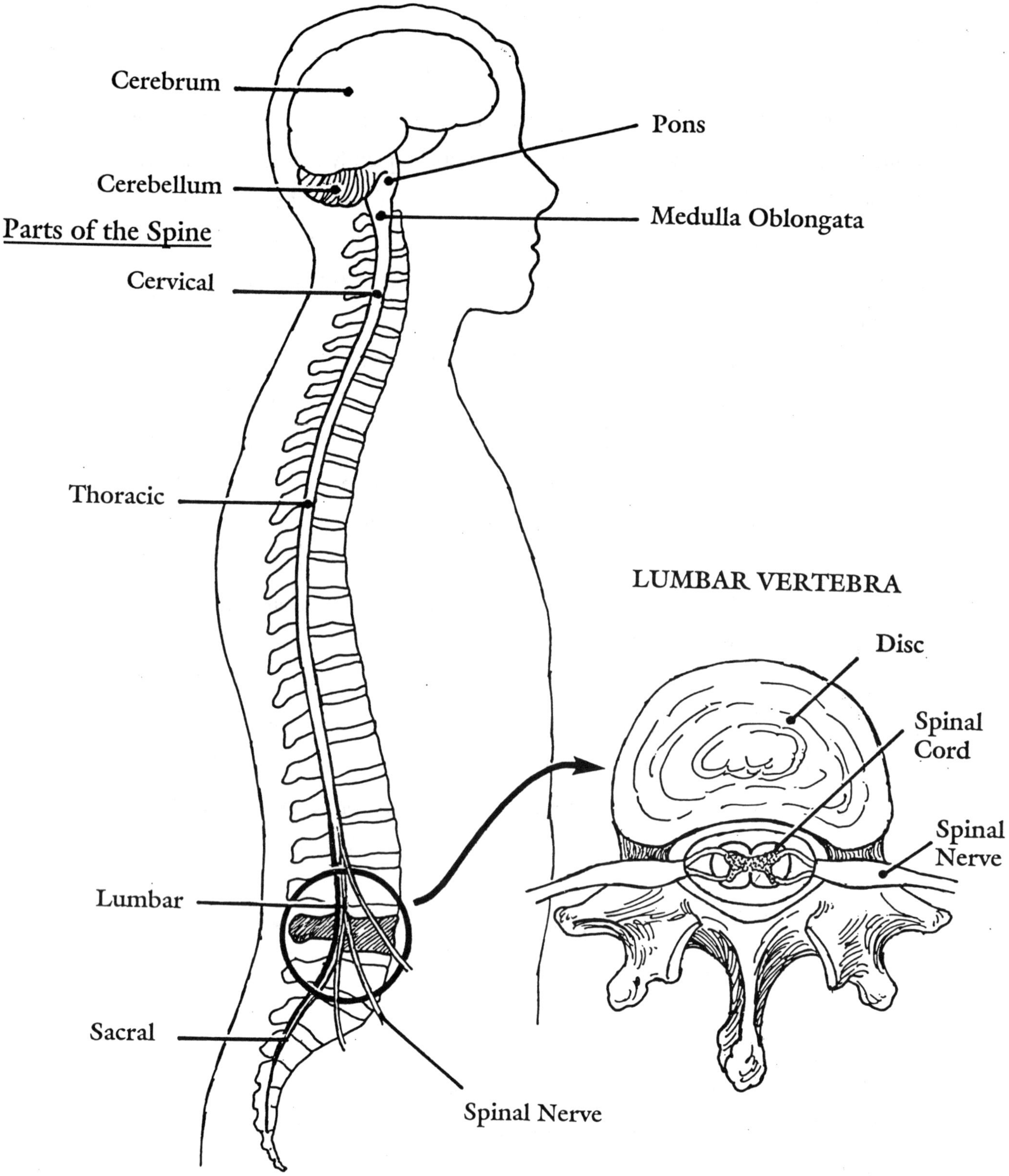

THE SPINAL CORD

Figure 12B

Types of sensory input that the brain receives from the trunk and limbs of the body and how they are tested:

a. Pain - a sensation which is unpleasant. This is tested by lightly pressing on an area of skin with a sharp object.

b. Temperature - distinguishing between hot and cold. This is tested by having a patient distinguish between hot and cold objects.

c. Pressure - a sensation of pressing down (such as the sensation of pressure on your feet while you are standing).

d. Simple touch - the sensation that you are being touched by something but not being able to define its size or shape. An example would be the sensation of being touched by a cotton swab.

e. Position sense - The sense of where a limb is positioned in relation to the rest of body. When catching a ball, for instance, your brain needs to know exactly where your hand is (without your having to look at it) so that it can control the movements necessary to get it directly in front of the ball. There are sensors in each muscle and joint that convey signals to the brain about exactly where each body part is located.

f. Fine touch - consists of being touched and being able to determine the size and shape of the object which is touching you. Doctors frequently use two pins placed a few millimeters apart and gently touch the patient with both at the same time. They ask the patient if they are being touched in one place or two. The closest distance between two pins at which the patient can recognize two sensations is an estimate of the fine touch capabilities of that area of skin. Different parts of the body have different abilities to perceive fine touch. The back, for example, is not as accurate as the tips of the fingers.

g. Vibratory sense - the feeling that something is vibrating. Doctors usually use the tuning fork for this test. While the fork vibrates they place it on one of the patient's joints and ask what is felt. The patient should describe vibration. Next, keeping the tuning fork in position, the doctor asks the patient to say as soon as the vibratory sensation stops. In general, the patient with normal vibratory nerve pathways should feel the vibration until it stops, or until the examiner with normal vibratory sense can no longer feel it.

Testing reflexes (so what's the hammer for?) :

Surely, almost everyone has had a doctor hammer on his or her arm or knee to "test the reflexes". If the reflex being tested is a true reflex, the brain does not control the movement, it happens automatically. When the doctor hammers on the tendon in front of the knee, which causes contraction of the quadriceps muscle, the message of muscle shortening travels to the spinal cord and immediately returns as an impulse through the nerves, making the lower leg jerk out forward.

Self demonstration:

You can demonstrate the knee reflex at home quite easily. Have someone sit on the edge of a table or bed with their legs dangling over the edge. They should be completely relaxed. Find their patellar tendon by feeling for the kneecap and the top of the shin bone. In the gap between these two bones, the tendon crosses the joint space of the knee. Now gently tap the tendon with a soft but firm object (a rubber spatula from the kitchen would be fine). Note the patellar reflex. Next, to exaggerate the effect of the output of the brain and spinal cord on the knee reflex, ask your subject to grab one hand in the other and try to pull his or her hands apart with all their strength. This extra motor output from the brain will exaggerate the knee reflex in such a way that it should be slightly more prominent if you test it while the subject is doing this hand-to-hand maneuver.

Abnormally brisk or dull reflexes indicate different problems. For example, if only one reflex or pair of reflexes are affected, it could mean that specific sensors, nerves, or muscles are diseased. If all the reflexes are abnormal, the whole spinal column or the brain could be diseased.

Each muscle in the body has a given strength depending on its use. Muscles that oppose gravity and move the entire body's weight are large and strong. Muscles that control fine intricate movements are smaller and weaker, such as the muscles of the hand. Doctors often test the strength of muscles or muscle groups by having a patient overcome forces applied against them. For example, the strength of the deltoid muscle (shoulder) could be tested by having the patient hold his or her arms straight out to the side, parallel to the ground, while the doctor tries to push the arms downwards toward the ground. The strength of the calf muscles may be tested by having the patient walk on his or her tip toes.

Testing the plantar response:

There is an additional reflex which should be tested for in any complete neurological exam. It is called the plantar response or Babinski test. This test is performed by stroking the sole of the foot with the edge of a rigid object (such as the handle of the reflex hammer) and observing the response of the big toe. Stroke the foot firmly, beginning near the heel and proceeding upwards along the outer edge of the foot and finally curving over towards the big toe. (Try this at home by using a key on the bottom of a volunteer's foot.) This stimulus is interpreted by the nervous system as a potentially dangerous one. The big toe curls downward to protect the sole of the foot by curving the bony structures of the foot upwards into an arch. Imagine stepping on a pin. As a reflex, your toes curl downward to prevent deep penetration of the pin and injury. This is a response similar to the plantar response. (This normal reflex is also controlled by the nerves in the brain and spine, in a way similar to the control of the knee jerk reflex, i.e. increased output increases the response, while decreased output inhibits the response.) In fact, with some diseases of the brain or spinal cord, the reflex is absent and the toe curls upward instead. Doctors call this a positive plantar response or Babinski sign and it indicates that there may be disease in the nervous system between the brain and the nerve tracts that send messages down the spine to control muscles. These problems may arise as a consequence of bleeding or tumors in the brain or spinal cord, or multiple sclerosis. The problems may also be due to metabolic imbalances such as: low glucose (sugar) in the blood, or low oxygen in the blood.

CHAPTER 13

The Skin

The largest organ of the body is, surprisingly, the skin. It has many important functions including protecting us from the extremes of temperature and weather, regulating the body's temperature, excreting wastes and water in the form of sweat, and, since it covers the whole body, it provides the brain with a sensitive surface to sense and respond to the environment. Doctors examine the skin because it can provide information to much of what may be going on inside the body.

The skin is examined using two of the doctor's primary methods of examination: observation and palpation.

The skin is made up of three layers: on the surface is a layer of mostly dead cells which are stacked up on one another. This layer is called the epidermis. The next layer is the dermis which lies just below the epidermis. It contains the structures which produce hair (follicles) as well as sebaceous glands which secrete sebum, a waxy, oily substance. The deepest layer of skin is the subcutaneous layer which contains fat, sweat glands and blood vessels.

Basic elements to examination of the skin:

1. Color: Melanin is a pigment in skin which determines its color. Individuals of different races have different skin colors based on the number of melanin cells in their skin which is genetically determined.

Indicators of illness may include pale skin which can be a sign of anemia (low numbers of red blood cells which carry oxygen). Mottled skin with alternating patches of pink and white in a net-like pattern is indicative of severe dehydration, or a lack of sufficient blood supply to the skin such as in shock.

In times of severe oxygen deficiency, skin can become blue in color. At other times skin may become yellow in color, as when patients have too much of a substance called bilirubin in their blood. Bilirubin is a substance formed when old red blood cells are broken down for recycling in the body. Too much bilirubin in the blood can be caused by too much breakdown of blood cells (such as in several blood and spleen diseases) or by slow processing of bilirubin in the liver.

The skin may also appear bronze in color, indicating difficulty with the body's ability to store iron or other elements such as copper.

The color of the skin does not in itself indicate a diagnosis, but points the doctor in the right direction to what may be going on.

2. Texture: The general feel of healthy normal skin is smooth, soft and somewhat moist. Doctors feel the skin to determine abnormalities in its texture. Rough skin, for example, can sometimes be a symptom of hypothyroidism, while velvet smooth skin may indicate hyperthyroidism.

3. Moisture: Skin conditions may be caused or made worse by the lack of moisture in the skin. Dry skin can indicate certain diseases such as hypothyroidism and allergic reactions.

4. Turgor: The turgor of the skin is a measure of its elasticity. If you take a pinch of a person's skin between your fingers and pull it up into a tent shape and then let go, you will notice that it will bounce back quite quickly, almost like rubber. But skin in a person that is severely dehydrated will not bounce back quickly. In fact, if the dehydration is severe, it may take several seconds for it to slowly resume its previous position. In addition, the skin of elderly people usually has less turgor since with aging it loses much of its elasticity.

5. Temperature: Since the skin is the largest organ of the body, it receives a larger proportion of the blood flow from the heart. The amount of blood flow to the skin is carefully controlled and is not a fixed percentage. The blood vessels which feed the skin can enlarge or constrict in such a way as to send more or less blood to the skin. When the body is hot, more blood is sent to the skin to produce sweat to allow for cooling. When the body is cool, blood is shifted away from the skin so that heat is not lost. In addition, when there is significant blood loss or dehydration the blood can flow from the skin to the vital organs such as the heart and brain. Thus the temperature of the skin is helpful in diagnosing medical problems.

6. Mucous membranes: Although not a part of the external surface of the body, mucous membranes (located under the eyelids, in the mouth and nose, in the vagina and rectum) can help determine the hydration status of the patient. A moist mouth is usually indicative of good hydration, while a dry mouth may indicate dehydration.

7. Lesions: Perhaps one of the most important parts of examining the skin is looking for lesions such as rashes, lumps, knots, or injured areas. These can be important clues to skin diseases as well as indications of diseases inside the body. For example, there are several changes which occur on the skin in certain places on the body when cancer is developing. These can serve as early signs to the doctor that cancer may be developing.

Doctors ask basic questions when confronted with abnormal skin areas: Questions, such as, "Is it flat or raised?" "Does it have smooth or irregular borders?" "What is its color?" "What is its texture?" "Does it have fluid or pus in it?" "What is its size?" "Where is it located on the body?" "Are there groups of lesions arranged in any particular way?" "Is it painful or does it itch?" The answers to all of these questions help in making an accurate diagnosis.

Skin Cancer:

Skin cancer is the most common type of cancer in the United States, and affects millions of people each year. It is important to diagnose early, since all types of skin cancer are curable if treated early enough. There are three main types of skin cancer, all related to sun exposure. People with fair skin who have been exposed to high levels of sun exposure and sunburn, (especially in the early years of life) are at higher risk for skin cancer.

Basal cell cancer: Appears as smooth and shiny raised lesions, sometimes with discoloration or visible blood vessels near the surface of the skin. This cancer rarely spreads to other parts of the body, but can be locally disfiguring.

Squamous cell cancer: Comprised of rough nodules with scabs or scales, which are often inflamed around the edges. Squamous cell cancer, like basal cell cancer, rarely spreads to the rest of the body, but sometimes it can. There is a higher risk of spread if the cancer is on the lip, temple, scalp, ears or genital areas.

Malignant melanoma: a dangerous kind of cancer of the pigment cells (melanocytes). This kind of cancer is the most deadly. After it spreads to other organs such as the liver, it is not considered curable. Caught early, the prognosis (outcome) depends on the depth of the tumor and whether or not it has spread. Melanomas are usually dark brown in color, darker than freckles. Some dark birthmarks have a risk of becoming melanomas, and should be watched closely for any of the changes that follow:

Signs of Malignant Melanoma:
Asymmetry: the lesion is not symmetrical
Borders are irregular
Color variegation: the color is different in different areas of the lesion.
Diameter: greater than 6mm
Elevation: above the skin surface

The most important rule for diagnosing all skin cancers is looking for change. If you have any areas which concern you, have someone look carefully at them and even note (draw) their size, shape and color. If they change over time, have a doctor look at them. Also, if a skin lesion is painful, itches, and bleeds, these can be early signs of a developing cancer.

The Appendages:

The skin has three main attachments or appendages: the hair, nails, and sweat glands.

1. Hair: The appearance of the hair can provide the doctor with medical information. There are several conditions that can affect the hair. Among these are lice, which can infest the hair, and some fungi which infect the skin of the scalp and hair follicles. These conditions are usually quite obvious and are easily treated. Hair loss is a common problem which affects some people. Hair loss is most frequently determined genetically, but is also related to age and gender. There are, however, several types of hair loss conditions that are related to skin diseases and certain stresses. Careful examination can help to distinguish the different causes of hair loss. In addition, certain metabolic diseases of the body such as hypothyroidism can cause hair loss.

2. Nails: Examination of the nails can be a clue to diseases also. Here are a few examples:

Clubbing: This is a condition in which the nails become dome-shaped instead of flat, and the angle between the nail and skin increases. This is caused by a long-term lack of oxygen in the tissues, and is commonly found in people with emphysema and lung cancer. It can also affect children with heart disease.

Pitting: These are small, crater-like pits in the nails. Commonly found in individuals having a skin disease called psoriasis.

Spooning: This occurs when there are not enough red blood cells circulating in the blood giving the nails a scooped-out or spoon-shaped appearance.

Beau's lines: are ridges which occur in the nail in a transverse direction. They are signs of recent severe illness. If for example, a person has a sudden severe illness and required hospitalization and even intensive care, the body, because of this great stress, can delay making good healthy nail tissue for several days (while it concentrates on other things). When the person recovers and normal nails begin to grow, a small ridge is left which represents the time of the acute illness.

Splinter Hemorrhages: These are small red/brown lines which run longitudinally along the nail. They represent areas of bleeding under the nail bed, and can occur when people have serious infections of their heart valves. When this happens, small infected pieces of the damaged heart valve can be broken off by the circulating blood, and travel downwards in the bloodstream. When they finally get trapped in a small vessel, (such as under the nail) they cause a small area of bleeding and infection. This bacterial infection of the inner surface of the heart and valves is called bacterial endocarditis. Manifestations of this same disease can cause changes in the palms and soles of the hands and feet as well as small areas of bleeding in the retina.

3. Sweat glands: These are found over most of the skin surface and secrete waste products and water in the form of sweat. These glands are not usually examined, since they are microscopic and buried under the skin. There is one test done in the laboratory which tests the composition of sweat for its content of chloride which is abnormal in persons with cystic fibrosis.

CHAPTER 14

Infection

Every tissue and organ of the human body can become infected with different living organisms. Infections are one of the leading causes for doctor visits and hospitalizations. The good news is that most infections are treatable and curable if caught early.

The Body's Response to Infection:

A. Temperature: Infections cause significant body changes. One such change is an elevation in the body temperature. This has two effects: it aids the body in fighting the infection, and causes the person with a fever to feel ill. High fevers can cause weakness, muscle aches, headaches, and other unpleasant symptoms.

Fever is useful in that it is an indicator that an infection may be present. There are, of course, many causes of elevated body temperature, but infection is by far the most common.

B. Lymph nodes: As blood flows out of the arteries to the capillaries which supply blood to individual tissues, most of it returns via the veins to the heart. Some proteins and cells, however, escape from the blood to bathe and nourish tissues. This fluid (lymph) does not re-enter the blood system directly, but instead migrates and flows through filters (the lymphatic system) before finally rejoining the circulatory systems at veins near the heart. The filters this fluid goes through are called lymph nodes. Lymph nodes are found throughout the body, like in the groin, armpits, neck, and behind the ears.

When a tissue is infected, signals are sent to the blood vessels which release more proteins and cells to bathe the tissue to help fight infection. When a lymph node becomes activated by an infection, it swells to several times its original size and often becomes palpable. Such lymph nodes are often tender, and when palpable, may signify infection.

There are, of course, other causes for enlarged lymph nodes, such as cancer. But again, infection is the most common cause of enlarged and tender lymph nodes.

C. Local signs of infection/inflammation: The body heals damaged or diseased tissue by causing an inflammatory response. Such responses bring cells and proteins to the damaged area to repair it. Inflammation is characterized by four signs and symptoms which are universally present wherever there is an infection:

Pain: When a tissue or organ is infected, the chemicals and proteins released by the inflammatory reaction cause pain. This pain is caused in part by the swelling that occurs, and in part by irritation of nerve endings.

Warmth: In the same way that the whole body can become fervish, the tissue at the site of infection becomes warm to touch.

Swelling: When infection is present, since more cells, proteins, and fluids are coming to the area to repair the tissue, it swells.

Redness: Blood flow to an infected area is increased when inflamed, so the area becomes reddened.

D. Bugs and drugs: There are four different classes of organisms which cause infection and they are treated differently.

Parasites: These are living organisms of different sizes which infect various body tissues and organs. They are unable to live alone outside the body since they derive their water and nutrition from the body. Many parasites have complicated life cycles in which they spend different stages of their life cycle inhabiting different animals. One specific malaria parasite, for example, spends part of its life cycle in the mosquito and the rest of its life cycle in the human bloodstream and liver.

Parasitic infections are usually diagnosed by signs and symptoms, but the diagnosis is often assisted by seeing the parasites directly under the microscope. This would occur, for example, in samples of stool, blood, or urine. Millions and millions of people are infected with parasites, most of them live in areas of poor sanitation, which makes the spread of parasites more likely. Fortunately, there are many effective drugs which treat and often cure almost all parasitic infections.

Bacteria: Bacteria are tiny unicellular organisms found throughout nature which can only be seen with a microscope. They live in the soil and in and on all plants and animals. Some are useful to the human body -- such as the bacteria which digest food in the intestines. Others live in and on the body without causing harm. Some, however, invade the tissues and cause dangerous and even life threatening infections. Bacteria are treated with antibiotics. However, certain antibiotics only kill certain bacteria.

When the infection is simple, the doctor can assume which bacteria are likely to be causing the problem and treat with an appropriate antibiotic. When an infection is unusual, serious, or life threatening, doctors like to know which bacteria are causing the infection and which antibiotics will kill them effectively. To find this out a small culture swab is placed in contact with the area of infection (whether that be the back of the throat, or in a deep wound) and sent to the laboratory. There it is placed in a specially designed material in which the bacteria will grow. Several days later colonies of bacteria which have grown can be tested chemically and identified under the microscope. This helps the doctor choose the appropriate antibiotic. Additional tests can be done to make sure that the antibiotic will be effective, since some bacteria develop resistance to antibiotics and are no longer destroyed by their use.

Viruses: Viruses are even smaller than bacteria. They have some, but not all the characteristics of living organisms. They reproduce, for example, but they do not grow or eat. Viruses reproduce by entering cells, hijacking them, and using their cellular processes to multiply. As a result the infected cells often die.

There are thousands of varieties of viruses and they cause many types of diseases. For example, the common cold, flu, warts, chicken pox, mumps, measles, and many gastrointestinal diseases are caused by viruses. Most viruses do not respond well to anti-viral medicines -- and most don't need to be treated since they run their course and the patient recovers. A few anti-virus medicines are effective for serious viral infections.

Fungi: These are organisms with a great variety of structures and form. Some, like bread mold are very small, while others like mushrooms are very large. Some types of fungi infect the human body, but most do not. Common human fungal infections include: athlete's foot, ringworm; some diaper rashes, and vaginal yeast infections in women.

NOTE TO READERS

If you like this book and you are interested in a special, custom-published version of the book individualized for your needs, or you would like a specific chapter developed into a brochure, please contact Kent Hughes at Harcourt Brace Custom Publishing, 301 Commerce Street, Suite 3700, Fort Worth, Texas 76102; Tel: (817) 334-7771; Fax: (817) 334-7880.

APPENDIX

Exercises: Practice What You've Learned

This activity is designed to demystify and acquaint students with the instruments found in the doctor's bag. A review of the introduction will be helpful in preparing to do this activity. It is recommended that the activity be conducted after the students have finished reading the entire text. The instruments for this activity can be purchased in any medical book store or medical supply house.

Students are not expected to become proficient in using the instruments in the doctor's bag. This is an introductory exercise intended to provide individuals with an appreciation for the information these instruments provide for doctors.

Six work areas, or stations may be set-up for this purpose. At each station an instrument is placed, students should follow the instructions listed below. Students are provided a work sheet to guide them through this activity. This activity is better conducted if students work in same sex pairs. Also, an evaluation sheet on the book and the unit of study is provided in this appendix.

For example, at station "1" a blood pressure cuff will be found. Students going to this station are provided with an opportunity to learn how a blood pressure is taken. One partner of a pair of students may have his or her blood pressure taken, while the other learns how to take a blood pressure. Partners then switch roles and repeat the activity.

At station "2" a reflex hammer is provided to enable students to learn about reflexes. The remaining four stations are set-up to follow the same format.

INSTRUCTIONS

The following instructions can be transcribed onto 8 1/2" x 11" sheets of paper and placed at each respective work station:

STATION 1: BLOOD PRESSURE STATION

- The blood pressure cuff measures the blood pressure in the arteries

systolic = pressure in arteries when heart is contracting

diastolic = pressure in arteries when heart is at rest

Normal blood pressure is around $\frac{120}{80}$

HOW TO TAKE SOMEONE'S BLOOD PRESSURE:

1. The subject should sit calmly for a few minutes.
2. Locate the brachial artery in the bend of the elbow with the arm straightened out.
3. Place the cuff around the upper right arm. (Make sure the arrow on the cuff is in line with the artery.)
4. Now feel the subject's radial pulse in his or her right wrist.
5. Make sure the air pump is closed and begin pumping the bulb attached to the cuff until you can't feel the pulse in the subject's wrist. Note the number on the gauge.
6. Release the air from the cuff.
7. Place the stethoscope in your ears and place the diaphragm (the larger diameter side) of the stethoscope over the brachial artery.
8. Now pump the cuff to 30 mm Hg above the number you saw on the gauge when the cuff blocked the artery.
9. Turn the screw valve slightly to allow the air out of the cuff slowly (2-5 mm Hg per second).
10. The number when you first hear a series of knocking sounds is the top number, or systolic blood pressure. The number you hear when the sounds disappear is the diastolic blood pressure, or bottom number.
11. Record the reading.

A patient may be considered to have high blood pressure if three consecutive diastolic pressures are found to be equal to or above 90 or when three consecutive systolic pressures are 140 or above.

STATION 2: REFLEX STATION

Reflex: A reflex is an involuntary response to a stimulus; a reflex action.

If only one reflex or pair of reflexes are abnormal, this may indicate that specific sensors, nerves, or muscles may be diseased. If all the reflexes are abnormal, the whole spinal column or brain may be diseased or altered by abnormal levels of hormones or chemical substances.

1. **Triceps reflex:** Have your partner allow his/her arm to hang loosely in a bent position (90 degrees at the elbow) while you hold their upper arm with one hand. Gently strike the triceps tendon with the reflex hammer, just above the elbow. Observe the reflex contraction of the triceps muscle (muscle on back of the upper arm).

2. Patellar reflex: Have your partner sit on a table with his or her feet dangling over the side, or have your partner cross one knee over the other while sitting down. Gently strike the patellar tendon just below the knee cap. Contraction of the quadriceps muscle (the large muscle in front of the thigh) causes extension of the lower leg.

3. Now to demonstrate the effect of the output of the brain and spinal cord, have the subject grab one hand in the other and try to pull his or her hands apart with all of his or her strength. This extra motor output from the brain will exaggerate the knee reflex in such a way that it should be slightly more prominent if you test it while your subject is doing this hand to hand maneuver.

STATION 3: HEART RATE STATION

Facts: The normal resting heart rate for most adults is about 72-80 beats per minute.
A newborn baby has a normal resting heart rate of 140-160 beats per minute.
A well-tuned athlete can have a resting heart rate of 50-60 beats per minute.

HOW TO TAKE THE HEART RATE (PULSE):

1. The easiest place to take the pulse is to feel for it on the wrist. Press your index and middle finger over the inside of the wrist (at the base of the thumb) until you feel a pulsation.
2. Count the number of beats you feel in one minute, or, count the number of beats in 15 seconds and multiply by 4 to get the rate per minute.
3. Take the resting pulse of your partner, then have them run up a stair case (or do jumping jacks), then take their pulse again. How does it compare?

If possible, see how caffeine affects the heart rate. Have someone drink a soft drink with caffeine in it. Do a before and after comparison. Any change?

Factors which increase heart rate:

Anxiety
Pain
Exercise
Hyperthyroidism
Anemia
Medications/drugs

Factors which decrease heart rate:

Sleep

Rest

Organic heart disorder

Hypothyroidism

Medications/drugs

STATION 4: EYE STATION

1. **The Snellen Eye Chart**

Purpose: To measure visual acuity

How: (1) Stand 20 feet from the eye chart and cover one eye with a 3x5 card. (2) With the uncovered eye, read aloud the smallest possible line of print. If you can read more than half of the letters in a given line, that is considered success for that line. (3) Cover the other eye and repeat the process.

What does it mean? (1) top number is the distance you are from the chart. (2) The bottom number is the distance at which the normal eye is able to read the letters on a given line on the chart.

Example: A 20/50 reading means that you see at 20 feet what the normal person sees at 50 feet.

20/20 is normal for each eye.

20/200 is legally blind.

Normal range is 20/20 - 20/40. After that, referrals are made.

2. **Pupillary Responses**

Pupil size is affected by the amount of light that enters the eye through the pupil (opening).

Increasing amounts of light cause the pupil to constrict; decreasing amounts of light cause the pupil to dilate (enlarge).

Penlight Test: Either go to a dark room or have your partner cup his or her hands over his or her eyes. Beam the pen light toward the side of one of the eyes, and gradually move it directly into the pupil. The pupil of the lighted eye should constrict as you move the light into it. Simultaneously, the opposite pupil should constrict.

STATION 5: HEART AND LUNG STATION

1. The Heart Sounds: Placing the diaphragm of the stethoscope over your partner's heart, listen for the normal "Lub-dupp-lub-dupp" sounds the heart makes. Doctors call these S1 and S2. The lub sound is actually the sound being made by the tricuspid and mitral valves of the heart when closing (the doors between the chambers of the heart on the right and left sides). The dupp sounds are the aortic and pulmonic valves closing (the doors at the exits to the right and left sides of the heart).

2. The Lung Sounds: Look (inspect) your partner's rate and depth of breathing. Count the respiratory rate or number of breaths in 30 seconds and multiply by 2. Inspect to see if both sides of the chest move together in symmetry.

3. Using the diaphragm of the stethoscope, listen to (auscultate) your partner's lungs both in front (anterior) and back (posterior). Can you hear the normal bronchial and vesicular sounds? The sounds heard are due to air moving freely through the airways in the lungs. The pitch and quality of these sounds are different, but they are normal and heard in most people.

Can you detect the difference between bronchial and vesicular breath sounds? The lower lobes of the lungs (toward the lower right and left sides of the back) are the best places to hear vesicular sounds. Have your partner inhale and exhale deeply to see if you can detect a difference between bronchial and vesicular sounds.

Would the breathing sounds of a person who smokes be different?

3. Feel (Palpate) your partner's chest to check for symmetry in breathing. Place your hands on the upper right and left sides of your partner's chest. As your partner inhales and exhales, does the chest expand evenly on either side? Ask your partner to say "ninety-nine". Are the vibrations felt equally in both hands?

STATION 6: HEARING STATION

1. **Weber Test:** Strike the tuning fork against the palm of your hand. Place the base of the tuning fork in the middle of your head. In which ear is the sound heard the loudest? It should be heard equally in both ears.

2. **Rinne Test:** Strike the tuning fork against the palm of your hand and place the stem of it on the mastoid bone directly behind the ear. When you stop hearing the tuning fork, reverse it and move the vibrating end of the fork to within one inch from the opening of your ear. Note when you stop hearing the hum. Normally, the sound is heard twice as long by air conduction than by bone conduction. Repeat the procedure on the other ear.

EXERCISE ACTIVITIES WORK SHEET

1. BLOOD PRESSURE STATION

What was your blood pressure? ____________________

What was your partner's blood pressure? ________________

2. REFLEX STATION

Were you able to get a triceps reflex?	YES	NO
Was the reflex equal in both arms?	YES	NO
Were you able to get a patellar reflex?	YES	NO
Was the reflex equal in both legs?	YES	NO

What impact did the hand-to-hand maneuver have on the patellar reflexes?

Why?

3. HEART RATE STATION

What was your resting heart rate? __________ beats per minute

What was your partner/s resting heart rate? ______________ bpm

What was your heart rate after you did 25 jumping jacks?

___________ beats per minute.

4. EYE STATION

What is your vision according to the Snellen Eye Chart?

Right Eye ______________

Left Eye _______________

Describe what you observed when you shined the pen light into your partner's eye? ______________________________

____

____

5. HEART and LUNG STATION

Were you able to hear your partner's heart beat? YES NO

What is making the first heart sound ("lub")? ______________________________

____

What is making the second heart sound ("dupp"?) ______________________________

____

Were you able to distinguish between bronchial and vesicular sounds in the lungs? YES NO

Please describe the sounds you heard. ______________________________

____

____

6. HEARING STATION

Describe the results of the Weber Test ______________________________

____

____

Describe the results of the Rinne Test ______________________________

____

____

EVALUATION OF THE BOOK AND UNIT OF STUDY ON THE PHYSICAL EXAM

Directions:

Please fill out the following evaluation and return this form to your instructor upon completion.

QUESTIONS ABOUT THE BOOK:

1. What are the strengths of the book? Why?

2. What are the weaknesses of the book? Why?

3. Which chapters/sections were particularly helpful? Which chapters/sections needed improvement? Why?

4. Was the book helpful (clear and informative)? Did you feel you learned more about your body than you knew before you had read the book?

5. Would you recommend the book to others?

QUESTIONS ABOUT LECTURE AND SMALL GROUP:

6. Please critique the lectures on the physical exam.

7. Please critique the small group lab experience.

OVERVIEW OF THE PHYSICAL EXAMINATION

(Outline of a demonstration lecture)

By Scott Isaacs, M.D.

1. **General Survey**

Briefly inspect patient for stature, habitus, sexual development, weight, posture, grooming, odors of body or breath, gait, speech and level of consciousness.

2. **Vital Signs**

Pulse - bradycardia or tachycardia; regular or irregular
Respirations - rate, depth, rhythm
Blood Pressure - hypotension or hypertension
Temperature - hyperthermia (fever) or hypothermia

3. HEENT (Head, Eyes, Ears, Nose, Throat)

Head - skull, scalp, face, sinuses
Eyes - visual acuity, visual fields, eyebrows, eyelids, lacrimal apparatus, conjunctiva, sclera, cornea, pupils, extraocular muscles, funduscopic exam
Ears - external ear, ear canal, tympanic membrane, hearing, Weber, Rinne
Nose - septum, mucosa, turbinates

Oral Pharynx - lips, buccal mucosa, gingiva, teeth, tongue, posterior oral pharynx, palate, tonsils

4. **Neck** - lymph nodes, thyroid, trachea, carotid artery, jugular vein

5. **Chest and Lungs** - inspection, palpation, percussion, auscultation

6. **Cardiovascular System** - inspection, palpation, auscultation (we do not usually percuss the heart)

7. **Arterial Pulses**

8. **The Breast Exam**

While in the sitting or standing position with arms at the sides ...**Inspection** - to note size, symmetry, contour, appearance of skin, and nipples. Raise arms above the head and again inspect paying special attention for dimpling or retraction. Place hands on hips and contract pectoralis muscles and again inspect. Next, lean forward looking for abnormalities. Examine the axillae (armpit), noting the condition of the skin. While relaxing with the arm down, cup together fingers and reach high into the axilla feeling for lymph nodes. Examine the breast in the sitting position. Next, lie down and place pillow under shoulder. Raise the arm (on side of breast to be examined) above head. Use pads of middle three fingers in rotary motion to compress tissue against chest wall. Proceed systematically, examining the entire breast. Do not forget the "tail" of breast. Finally, palpate nipple and areola, noting discharge or retractions.

9. **Abdomen** - inspection, auscultate, percuss, palpate (liver, spleen, aorta, masses)

10. **Male Genitalia**

Inguinal Area - lymph nodes, hernias

Scrotum and Testes - between thumb and first two fingers, palpate each testis and epididymis. Note size, shape, consistency and tenderness. Note any new masses or irregular areas. Identify spermatic cord and palpate between thumb and fingers.

Penis - look for ulcers, scars and discharge

11. **Female Genitalia** - inspection, speculum exam, bimanual exam, pap smear, wet prep.

12. **Musculoskeletal Exam** - joints, tendons, ligaments, bursae, muscles

13. **Neurological Exam** - level of consciousness, higher cognitive abilities, cranial nerves, sensations, motor strength, coordination, deep tendon reflexes, gait.

14. **Skin** - texture, rashes, scars, edema

15. **Rectal exam**

EXAMINATION OF THE CRANIAL NERVES

(A More Detailed Discussion as an Extension of Chapter 11)

There are twelve pairs of cranial nerves. The nerves which branch out directly from under the brain are called the cranial nerves. Doctors frequently examine cranial nerves with simple tests to determine that they are all intact and functioning correctly. The following describes the way the doctor evaluates the functioning of these nerves **(See Figure Appendix 1):**

Cranial Nerves Pair #1: The olfactory nerves (smelling):

These nerves enter the skull at the very top of the nasal cavity, and provide us with the sense of smell. This pair is usually checked by presenting the patient with aromas from small jars containing some common and distinctly smelling items such as coffee, soap or cinnamon.

Cranial Nerve Pair #2: The Optic Nerves (seeing):

The optic nerves originate in the retina of the eye and exit the eyeball at the very back where they enter the brain. Their function is tested in two primary ways: In the first the patient is administered the well-known Snellen eye chart test -- that's the one with the big "E" where you have to read the letters down to as small as you can see them. This test examines visual acuity.

In the second, the doctor tests peripheral vision -- that's the area of vision which sees things off to the side of where a person is actually focusing their eyes.

The light reflecting off this page, for example, is entering your eye, and being focused on the center of your retina. Off to the side, however, you can see other things, such as the rest of the room in which you are sitting. These things are being seen by the outer part of the retina and are in your peripheral vision. Doctors can test this in many ways and with various instruments, but here is a simple test you can try on your own.

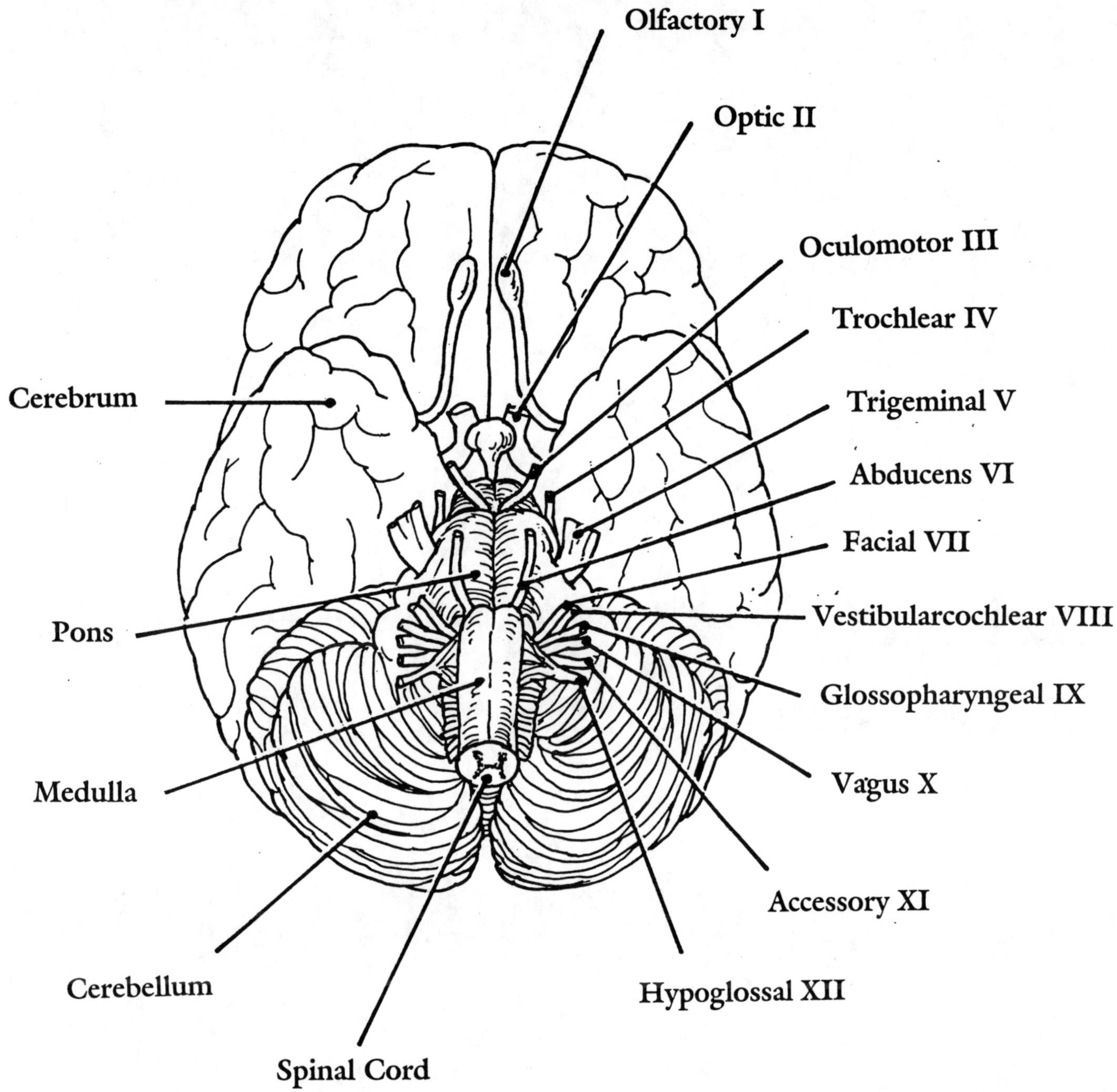

BASAL VIEW OF BRAIN AND CRANIAL NERVES

Figure Appendix 1

Have someone look you straight in the face at a distance of about three feet, and ask them to focus on your nose. Place your hands up into the air to the left and right, midway between your face and theirs. Hold up two or three fingers and ask them how many fingers they see. If they can tell how many fingers there are without taking their focus off your nose, then you can be reasonably sure that the upper peripheral vision works on both sides. Move your hands to below the level of their eyes, and change the number of fingers you are holding up on both sides. Now you are testing the lower right and left peripheral fields of vision.

There are six muscles that move each eye. These muscles are intricately controlled and coordinated by three pairs of cranial nerves (nerves 3, 4 and 6) which allow the eye to move in its socket to follow moving objects, stay focused on one object while the head moves, and keep both eyes on the same object. If this system fails, we see double, or are unable to track moving objects and/or keep our eyes fixed on an object while our head is moving.

Cranial nerve Pair #3 (oculomotor nerves):

This pair of nerves functions to move the muscles which cause the eye to move upward, downward, and inward.

This nerve pair also carries fibers from the sympathetic and parasympathetic nervous systems which control the muscles which focus the lens of the eye for near and far vision. They also control the muscles which adjust the size of the pupil to let the correct amount of light into the eyes, similar to the aperture of a camera. When the room is dark the pupil gets bigger to let more light in; when the room is bright, the pupil gets smaller to let less light in.

Cranial Nerve Pair #4 (trochlear nerves):

These nerves control the muscles which move the eyeball downward and inward at the same time.

Cranial Nerve Pair #5 (trigeminal nerve):

These nerves have two primary functions. The first is to control the main muscles of chewing. If you clench your teeth tightly together as if you were trying to grind a big piece of steak, you can feel a muscle on either side of your face (in your cheeks) contract to pull your jaws together. These are two muscles controlled by the fifth nerve pair. Doctors test this by asking you to bite down hard and then feeling the muscles to see that they are well contracted on both sides.

The second function of the fifth nerve pair is to convey sensation to the brain. This sensation (or sense of touch) comes from the skin of much of the head (especially the face), the outer surface of the eardrum, the sinuses and the membrane which surrounds the brain.

Cranial Nerve Pair #6 (abducens nerves):

This pair of nerves moves the muscle on the outer side of the eyeball which allows the eye to look toward the side.

The simplest way to test the correct operation of all the nerves that move the eyes is to have the patient move their eyes in the shape of an "H" while following the doctor's moving finger. If the eyes have difficulty moving in one of those directions, the doctor can figure out which muscle is not working and, hence, which nerve is dysfunctional.

Cranial Nerve Pair #7 (facial):

The facial nerve pair is quite complex and has four main functions:

1. It provides the muscles of facial expression with control. These muscles control such things as smiling, frowning, closing the eyes, winking, raising the eyebrows and other such helpful nonverbal human expressions.
2. It provides nerve supply to most of the glands of the head, such as the salivary glands and the tear glands.
3. It provides a small area of skin around the outside of the ear with the sense of touch.
4. It provides the sense of taste to the front two-thirds of the tongue.

This nerve pair is usually tested in a simple way by asking the patient to make certain facial expressions, such as smiling or closing their eyes very tightly. Some patients who have had a stroke, for example, are unable to close their eyes completely, or can only close them weakly and are unable to keep them closed while they are gently pried open. This nerve pair can further be tested more completely and formally by challenging a patient with certain tastes and seeing if they are recognized. However, if there is no complaint by the patient about tasting difficulty then this test is not usually necessary.

Cranial Nerve Pair #8 (vestibulocohlear):

This pair of nerves has two functions. The first is related to balance. In the inner ear, which is responsible for balance, there are three circular canals which are fluid filled and which are oriented in three directions (up and down, left and right, and front and back). When the head moves, the brain can figure out in which direction the movement has occurred by calculating in which direction the fluid in the canals has moved. When the system malfunctions or is diseased a person becomes unsteady in their manner of walking and often becomes dizzy, or may feel as if the room is spinning around them (vertigo).

The second function of the eighth pair of cranial nerves is hearing. The nerves transmit sound from the middle and inner ear (where it is received and encoded) to the brain (where it is interpreted). Hearing can be formally tested by checking each ear for hearing at different frequencies and volumes. Usually just demonstrating that a person can hear a faint whisper is sufficient to demonstrate that this pair of nerves is intact.

Cranial Nerve Pair #9 (glossopharyngeal):

This nerve pair has the following functions:

1. Supplies nerve stimulation to a single muscle in the throat.

2. Provides intervention to the parotid glands which are located in front of each ear. These glands secrete saliva which helps in the early stages of food digestion.

3. Senses the blood pressure in the carotid arteries of the neck, and also the carbon

dioxide content in the blood.
4. Provides the back one-third of the tongue with the sense of touch and taste. And also provides the inner side of the eardrum with the sense of touch.

Cranial Nerve Pair #10 (vagus):

The vagus nerve pair is the longest cranial nerve and has four main functions:
1. They provide connections (impulses) to the throat and voice box (larynx) to allow movement of these structures. Tests of this pair of nerves assure normal speech patterns and swallowing. In patients who are unconscious, its function can be tested by tickling the back of the throat with a cotton swab and seeing if the patient gags in response.
2. These nerves also provide nerve stimuli to the throat, voice box, heart, lungs, and abdomen. For example, the peristalsis motion of the gut in digesting food is controlled through the vagus nerves. In addition, the heart rate is in part controlled by the amount of stimulation it receives from the vagus nerves. Sometimes when the vagus nerves are over-stimulated by the brain (such as in conditions of extreme pain or emotional distress) the heart can slow down so much as to cause a person to faint.
3. They convey sensory information from the throat, voice box, and the abdominal and thoracic organs. For example, when the stomach becomes over-distended with food, the sensation of nausea that occurs has traveled to the brain through the vagus nerves.
4. Finally, they allow for a small area of the ear to be able to sense touch, temperature and pain.

Cranial Nerve Pair #11 (Accessory):

The accessory nerve pair has only one function. It supplies the nerves which move two muscles in the neck. The first is the trapezius, which is the bulky muscle to the back of the neck on either side which becomes particularly prominent in body builders. The second is the sternomastoid which, as the name suggests, connects the breastbone (sternum) to the mastoid process behind the ear. The function of the first muscle is tested by having the patient shrug her or his shoulders and noting that the movement is

symmetrical, while the sternomastoid muscle is tested by having the patient move her or his chin as far as possible toward the left or right against a resisting force. Try the latter test in front of a mirror and you will see the front of your neck flatten and the sternomastoid muscle contract.

Cranial Nerve Pair #12 (hypoglossal):

This nerve pair controls the movement of the tongue. The muscles inside the tongue serve to make it wide or thin, flat or thick, while the muscles outside the tongue serve to move the tongue in and out of the mouth and from side to side. Doctors usually test this nerve pair by having the patient stick his/her tongue out of the mouth.